Shuffle On: Never Quit or Say You're Done

Wendall Woodall

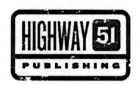

Highway 51 Publishing, LLC
Mint Hill, North Carolina
HWY51.com

Published by Highway 51 Publishing, LLC
Mint Hill, North Carolina
HWY51.com

ISBN: 0-9960570-6-4
ISBN-13: 978-0-9960570-6-6

Library of Congress Control Number: 2016958925

Cover design: Steven Mast, Mast Design
Editing: Kristen Driscoll, Highway 51 Publishing

Praise for *Shuffle On: Never Quit or Say You're Done*

"I just finished reading *Shuffle On: Never Quit or Say You're Done*, by Wendall Woodall. It is truly an inspiration for those who are afflicted with Parkinson's disease. But it is more than that. Brutally honest, yet brimming with faith, hope, and love, it is an inspiration for all of us."

Diane Rivers
Chair of the Board
Parkinson Association of the Carolinas

"Windy has done it again! With deep compassion and empathy, he provides readers with keen insights and biblical encouragement. His years of pastoral leadership and heart for God are so evident as he gives practical help and inspiration to anyone struggling with challenges in life."

Michael T. Boulware
Campus Pastor
Forest Hill Church • Waxhaw, North Carolina

To all the Movement Disorder Specialists out there:
Thank you for helping us *shuffle on*!

Contents

Preface 1

Waiting 5

Wiring 19

Weeping 35

Why-ing Part 1 53

Why-ing Part 2 71

Writing 87

Working 101

Winning 117

Acknowledgments 133

Preface

In my first book, *Shuffle*, I wrote about my first thousand days after being diagnosed with young onset Parkinson's disease. I know, I know. I still like to mention that "young" part every chance I get, don't I? As someone pointed out to me the other day, Parkinson's is Parkinson's. You either have it or you don't. Of course, she might have just been upset that she couldn't use the phrase "young onset" with hers. I tried not to gloat.

The story of my first thousand days took me from August 18, 2011, the day I received the diagnosis, until mid-May 2014. As I write these words, I'm now a full year into my second thousand days with Parkinson's. Somehow, it just felt like I was overdue for a sequel. Besides, a lot more history has been written since that first book. My friend, Vince, and I did restart that local support group for people with Parkinson's and their caregivers, and we've been going strong for well over a year now. We meet the second Monday of every month at a local YMCA. It's an impressive gathering of some pretty awesome people, and I'm not just saying that because I know they will read these words.

I finally decided to undergo the deep brain stimulation

(DBS) surgery, which was a fascinating experience. I'll give more details in chapter two. On the day of the surgery, I taped a note for the neurosurgeon to the top of my head. It read: "Hey, Doc, be very, very careful when you start to drill here. Just saying!" It was either that or, "Call before you dig." I went with the first one, and, evidently, he was careful, for which I am deeply appreciative. Pun intended.

Along the way, I've been trying to start a movement. That's right, a movement, complete with a cool catchphrase and inspirational theme song. No biggie. For the catchphrase, I went back to my childhood. As readers of my first book will know, I hail originally from the great state of Alabama, home of the Crimson Tide. There's a greeting we often use there that both the fans and the haters will recognize. I say a "greeting," but it's more of a greeting/salutation/welcome/good-bye/send-off/blessing/prayer/all-purpose verbal exchange in which just two words are spoken. You probably know them, whether you are a football fan or not. So, say them with me, just this one time: *Roll Tide!* See how easy that was! It's simple, effective, and packs a punch all at the same time. It's perfect.

Well, I wanted a phrase just like that one for all of us who have Parkinson's, an expression we could use either to greet or to take our leave of one another, and versatile enough to say to both friends and strangers. It would have to be something inspiring, with just a hint of a friendly challenge built in. And, while the two-word phrase I came up with may not ever be as well known as *Roll Tide!* ... it's got great potential. It's simply this: "Shuffle on!" I end almost every meeting or talk with those two words: "Shuffle on!" I hope to make it even better known through the distribution of this book. The accompanying fist bump could be optional, of course, for reasons obvious to those of us with Parkinson's.

Thus, with the catchphrase in place, only the theme song was missing. For inspiration, I turned once again to my childhood, and one song quickly rose to the top of the charts, as it had when I was a teenager. The year was 1976, and the band was Kansas. The song was a last minute addition to the album, but as soon as the band heard it, they knew it would be the lead track—and they were right. The song, "Carry On Wayward Son," was their first major hit, the one that made them famous. I'll bet you can just hear that great *a capella* intro even now, am I right? It's still one of those sing-at-the-top-of-your-lungs songs every time it airs on the radio.

Well, with sincere apologies to Kerry Livgren and Kansas, I tweaked the words just a bit for those of us with Parkinson's, and the result was a thing of beauty, if I do say so myself. Get that *a capella* tune going in your head and then sing these words:

> Shuffle on with Parkinson's
> Never quit or say you're done
> When you need to, take a rest
> Then, won't you try once more?

OK, remember: Beauty is in the eye—or ear—of the beholder! But don't brush it aside too quickly. It's kind of catchy once you start singing the new lyrics over and over again. In fact, the words will get stuck in your head, and that's what theme songs are supposed to do, right?

These words have become the anthem of my second thousand days. They voice the message at the core of this movement I want to start, even if that only extends as far as my own local support group. The crux of the message is this: No matter what may come our way, we will never quit or say we're done. Instead, we will shuffle on! And we'll keep on shuffling until we can shuffle no more.

Oh, and one more thing: We will bring along as many fellow shufflers as we possibly can! Fist bump, miss. Fist bump, miss. Oh, never mind. Just ... shuffle on!

Wendall "Windy" Woodall
Charlotte, North Carolina

Chapter One
Waiting

Why do you stand here looking into the sky? —Acts 1:11

Most of us either grew up reading or raised our children reading the best-selling children's books by Dr. Seuss. I'm sure we all had our favorites. Mine included such classics as, *Horton Hears a Who*, *The Cat in the Hat*, *Green Eggs and Ham*, and *One Fish Two Fish Red Fish Blue Fish*—all titles dating back to the 1950s and 1960s. However, in 1990, just a year before he died, Theodor Geisel pulled off the impossible. He published one more book, one that has since become, arguably, the most popular of them all. It was called *Oh, the Places You'll Go!*

The children who received the book that first year—and in the years that followed—absolutely loved it, and it became yet another Dr. Seuss story to be read again and again. An instant classic! The interesting fact about the book, however, is that it also turned out to be quite legendary among teenagers and twentysomethings. How did that happen? Well, I'm not sure who started the trend, but *Oh, the Places You'll Go!* quickly became a popular book to give as a high school or college graduation gift. Today, thousands of copies are sold during the yearly graduation season. And, let's face it, it's a much more interesting gift than the usual suspects: engraved pen and pencil sets and monogrammed luggage pieces.

I like the book because it's a fairly accurate description of life. The star of the story, a little man dressed in a one-piece yellow jumpsuit and toboggan, starts out with great enthusiasm—as we all do, right? He tries to choose the right paths and make all the right decisions. He ends up experiencing victories and setbacks, the highest heights and the lowest slumps, ultimate fame and extreme loneliness. Eventually, as he faces up to his problems and keeps moving forward despite the obstacles, he finds success.

It's not a happy-ever-after ending, the kind of ending which I tend to reject because it's not the kind of life that most people actually experience. I'd much rather have a little reality blended into the story, and Dr. Seuss does just that. The protagonist has to keep moving and invest a bit of his own blood, sweat, and tears to make it to the end. That's real life! Sometimes, it seems as if we're taking three steps forward, two steps back, but we hope we're always making progress toward a better future.

At this point, you must be asking yourself: *Why are we still talking about a children's book?* Because, as is the case so often with Dr. Seuss, his words are not directed only toward his young readers, but to all who are passing through this experience called life. And one of the most ominous places he describes in the whole book is not, as you might suspect, where the weather is foul, where our enemies prowl, or even where the Hakken-Kraks howl. It's a place he simply refers to as "The Waiting Place." I happen to think it's the scariest scene. Every face is sad. Every pair of eyes is closed or staring blankly into nothingness. No one is moving; no one is working; and no one is doing anything but waiting. On what were they waiting? Trains, planes, buses, mail, phone calls, a change in the weather, their hair to grow, or water to boil. Dr. Seuss, of course, made it all rhyme. These were all tangible things, but he listed some intangible things as well, like a yes or no answer or a better break or another chance. A few people on this page of his book look mad. Some look asleep. Most look like they're in a trance from the sheer boredom of waiting. Do you know what I see on this page? I see people who have either given up or who simply got tired of trying. Their circumstances were too much for them, so they decided to sit down, or lie down, and wait. What are they waiting for, exactly? They're waiting for something about their circumstances to change on its own.

Instead of getting up and attempting to make some things happen—creating, if you will, their own better break or another chance—everyone on this page has chosen to stop indefinitely and wait. Uselessly, I might add. How do I know it's all for naught? Because—spoiler alert—I've read the entire book from cover to cover, multiple times, and the ending never changes. The fellow in yellow makes it! But none of these wait-ers ever gets the things he or she is waiting for. Go look for yourself! The wait-ers are still there, stuck forever on the same page.

The older and wiser Geisel, well into his eighties when he published this story, on the very next page yells his advice to Mr. Yellow and the readers: "NO!" he shouts. "That's not for you!" Somehow find a way to escape all that waiting and staying, he says. Somehow get away from that most useless place: the waiting place.

~

Let's face it. When it comes to Parkinson's, there have

been moments when I had to just sit and wait, but I hated every minute of it. Scheduling my first appointment with a general neurologist—and then with a movement disorder specialist—had me waiting for weeks. The time seemed to go agonizingly slowly, no doubt because I wanted all the answers immediately. Doctors have incredibly busy schedules, I know, and they can only add so many new patients a year. Later, I learned that I was somewhat lucky that it was only weeks for me. I have friends who wait four to six months just to get in the office door for their initial consultations. That's a long time to wait, especially if there's every indication that the news is probably going to be devastating.

The worst part of my DBS surgery was the time I had to wait between the different phases. When phase one was completed, I had to wait eight days for phase two. It was nine days between phases two and three, and twelve days between phases three and four. It almost killed me. When you're sitting around waiting for the day the neurosurgeon will drill holes in your newly shaved and up-to-now scar-free skull, it can produce some anxiety, to say the least. The longer you wait, the more time on your hands to worry and fret and contemplate worst-case scenarios. At least, that's what I've heard. I experienced none (OK, how about all?) of those feelings, myself.

Of course, there are unavoidable times when others require us to wait and we have no say-so. However, when we do get to be part of the decision-making process, we should vote to get up, get going, and avoid the useless waiting as much as we can. As far as I'm concerned, praying for a miracle from God and/or hoping that modern medicine will one day discover a cure is not time wasted, either. Sometimes, such actions of faith are our only guardrails against despair. But, in that space between the miracle and today or between the cure and today—in that meantime, if you will—we need to be helping things along. I call those actions of faith, too.

I've heard it said that we should pray as if everything depended on God, and then work as if everything depended on us. In my personal faith, I believe the former more than the latter, but I'll never stop doing both.

Let me give you a living, breathing example. Recently, when I was attending a book signing, my wife and I met a woman with Parkinson's. Irene was 82 years old. She was sporting a beautiful green pantsuit, which looked perfect with her bright red hair. She kept saying that I was too young to have Parkinson's, so I liked her from the start. The funny thing, though, was that I had the same thought about her. Maybe that was because she told us that she had just been skydiving for the first time in her life.

"Why would you do that?" my wife, Cheryl, kept asking her. "Why would you jump out of a perfectly good airplane?"

"Because I had never done it before," Irene said. Later, we coaxed out of her that she might have been influenced to go through with it because of the handsome young man to whom she had been assigned for her first tandem jump. Your first jump is always tandem.

Anyway, what I love about Irene is that she didn't watch life pass by her. She didn't sit around waiting. She created her own better breaks. The eye candy on her arm and the dopamine rush she must have felt on her way down would have been a good start.

~

Now, allow me to return to the verse that opens this chapter and give you fair warning about the chapters to come. As in my former book, I try to connect a theme verse or Bible passage with the content of each chapter. Ideally, the connection is already there, and I'm just pointing out the obvious. Sometimes, only a look at the context—the grammatical, historical, linguistic, and cultural context in which the verse is originally found—will reveal that connection. Other times, only a look at all of the above by a more experienced and qualified scholar and theologian will do. Sometimes ... well, let's just hope for the obvious more often than not.

You may be wondering: *Why look for the meaning of a scripture at all?* The quick answer is that I have found that biblical truths and principles are worth living by. I believe in God and his son, Jesus Christ, and I am a follower of Christ. This means that I am attempting to follow his lead in my life with regard to both his teachings and his actions. It means that I extend grace both to myself and to others when I, or they, don't get it right. Do you have to be a follower of Christ in order to live by the biblical truths and principles found in God's Word? Not necessarily, but he does serve as a great motivational figure. All that to say, you can skip over these spiritual parts of the book if you want, but I think it would be worth it to at least hear out these truths and then make your decision. You might be pleasantly surprised at how relevant the Bible is.

Now, back to Acts chapter 1. One of the first things you should ask about the context is: Who was the author? In this case, it's Luke, the same guy who wrote the Gospel of Luke and the only non-Jewish (or Gentile) writer in the New Testament, which is significant. Most of the early converts to Christianity were Jewish. The fact that they accepted this book as part of the New Testament is incredible given the fact that Luke was both non-Jewish and a non-apostle. Luke was a doctor, which tended to give him an eye or ear for detail and made him a very careful investigator; he liked things put in order, and that's probably why he made such a good historian. He was most likely Paul's convert and became a fellow traveler and, no doubt, a supporter of Paul's ministry—not to mention his unofficial biographer.

The book of Acts covers the first thirty years after the Ascension of Christ, which is exactly where Acts 1 drops us off—or him off. Jesus has just ascended to heaven and the disciples are hoping for one last glimpse of him.

> After he said this, he was taken up before their very eyes, and a cloud hid him from their sight. They were looking intently up into the sky as he was going, when suddenly two men dressed in white stood beside them. "Men of Galilee," they said, "why do you stand here looking into the sky? This same Jesus, who has been taken from you into heaven, will come back in the same way you have seen him go into heaven (Acts 1:9-11).

If ever you wanted a cloudless day, this would have been it! But these guys weren't giving up hope! They were looking *intently*—no distractions—which is evident by what took place next.

Suddenly, out of nowhere, Luke tells us, two men dressed in white (that's code for angels) were standing beside them. And when that in itself wasn't enough to get their attention, the angels spoke to them: "Men of Galilee, why do you stand here looking into the sky?"

We have to give the disciples a break here. They were not functioning at full capacity. They had just seen what had to be one of the strangest things they had witnessed in all their time with Jesus. The Bible merely says that Jesus was taken up before their very eyes up into the clouds. I've often wondered if that was like a helium balloon being released into the sky, you know, slow and steady with wind drifts slightly affecting his course. Or I wonder if he assumed the position for takeoff, and, with one hand lifted skyward and the other fisted tightly by his side, speak the first version of the now cliché phrase, "Up, up, and away!" The latter would have been cooler, of course, but the former is probably closer to what really happened.

There is only one other ascension recorded in the Bible. His name was Elijah and, by all appearances, his was much more attention-grabbing than the one described in Acts.

> As they were walking along and talking together, suddenly a chariot of fire and horses of fire appeared and separated the two of them, and Elijah went up to heaven in a whirlwind. Elisha saw this and cried out, "My father! My father! The chariots and horsemen of Israel!" And Elisha saw him no more (2 Kings 2:11-12).

Elijah was swept up by chariots of fire, pulled by horses of fire, with a whirlwind to boot! It doesn't get much more exciting than that. But then again, everything about Jesus' first coming seemed to be planned with low-key in mind. He was born in a manger in the little town called Bethlehem. His family came from the can-anything-good-come-from-there village of Nazareth. He had an uneventful childhood, and his miracles were often followed by orders not to tell anyone. He never traveled more than 200 miles from his hometown. His unfair trial took place at night. He was crucified between two common thieves, buried in a borrowed tomb, and appeared mainly to his disciples after his resurrection. Then, he ascended quietly and unheralded back to heaven with no chariots of fire or even the theme music from the movie, which would have been at least something.

But the angels do make a promise: "This same Jesus, who has been taken from you into heaven, will come back in the same way you have seen him go into heaven." He came in obscurity the first time. For his second appearance, it seems there might be a little more fanfare:

> Then will appear the sign of the Son of Man in heaven. And then all the peoples of the earth will mourn when they see the Son of Man coming on the clouds of heaven, with power and great glory (Matthew 24:30).

All the peoples of the earth will see him the second time around. I think there are even rumors of a trumpet call of God. Who knew God played the trumpet?

But there's something else I want you to see about the angels' question in this passage. Yes, there's a promise of a second coming, but look back at Acts 1:7-8. The disciples are asking about the timing, and this is how Jesus responds:

> It is not for you to know the times or dates the Father has set by his own authority. But you will receive power when the Holy Spirit comes on you; and you will be my witnesses in Jerusalem, and in all Judea and Samaria, and to the ends of the earth (Acts 1:7-8).

Did you catch this? Jesus had left them a task to do—to be the eyewitnesses of all the events of his life and ministry in ever-widening geographical circles. The task would eventually lead all but one to a martyr's death. As soon as Jesus had spoken these words, Luke tells us, he was taken up before their very eyes.

Now, come back around with me and read the angels' question once more, this time with those parting instructions from Jesus still ringing in your ears, then tell me what you hear in their words: "Men of Galilee, why do you stand here looking into the sky?"

Do you know what I hear? My paraphrase would be this: "What are you guys still doing here? Isn't there something more important you should be doing, instead?" To which, the disciples all probably started talking at once, saying, "Oh yeah, right away!" and scrambling to get their things together and start walking back to Jerusalem, from where everything would commence.

I'm not sure if this story is purely legend, but, supposedly, someone asked Pope John XXII what he would say to the worldwide church if he knew that Jesus was going to return to earth the very next day. Allegedly, the pope flicked his hands in a kind of shooing motion and said, "Look busy!"

That's the scene I have in my mind when the angels ask the disciples this question. I can hear Peter barking out the orders, perhaps with the theme from *Madagascar* booming in the background: "Come on, guys. We got to Move it! Move It!"

~

We recently celebrated our second annual Parkinson's Awareness Walk hosted by the Parkinson Association of the Carolinas (PAC), and it was a great success. We called it the "Move It! Parkinson's Awareness Walk," or a shorter version, the "Move It! Walk." We did that for several reasons. First, exercise is the only clinically proven neuroprotective treatment for Parkinson's. That is, it's the only treatment that has been shown to slow down the progression of the disease. That is huge! Everything else is just symptoms management. So, when we give people the opportunity of walking instead of uselessly waiting, of staying active and engaged instead of just isolating themselves from everything and everyone else, then we are *Moving it! Moving it!* in the right direction.

In the team captain meetings leading up to the walk, we sort of poked fun at the fact that so many people with Parkinson's were actually going to be participating in the walk itself. *Bradykinesia*, or slowness of movement, is one of the four main symptoms of Parkinson's—they're the shufflers, if you will. With so many shufflers at the walk, we asked wouldn't this be the slowest walk in the history of our city? But our walk was not about going a specific distance. It was about each participant doing their very best—shufflers, non-shufflers and everyone in between— and feeling great about every step or shuffle they took to raise awareness about the disease itself and about a great organization (PAC) working to serve those affected by Parkinson's.

All in all, it was a wonderful day. It had rained the night before, but the day dawned bright and beautiful with a Carolina-blue sky, as we like to say in this part of the world. There was a proclamation from the mayor and the governor, both proclaiming April National Parkinson's Awareness Month. Sir Purr himself, the Carolina Panthers' mascot, was there, rooting everyone along, and the drum line from a local high school played to keep us marching on beat. There were even rumors of a devilishly handsome young grandson with a sign on his back, "In Honor of Papa," making quick time around the track, mostly splashing in the leftover puddles, but also riding on his

Papa's shoulders, yelling, "We win, Papa! We win!" We do indeed, Elisha, we do indeed.

~

With the verse I looked at a little earlier, I'm not suggesting that we all get involved in Christian ministry as a way of not getting stuck in that most useless place, The Waiting Place. I know that people with Parkinson's come from a wide variety of faiths and worldviews. I'm speaking from the Christian tradition, but whatever your tradition, I am sure it offers a wide variety of good suggestions, perhaps even commands, challenging you to find better things to do with your time than just standing around looking up intently into the sky.

If we can go back to Dr. Seuss, I am suggesting that instead of waiting around for a yes or no, or a better break or another chance, we simply ought to be out doing those things that bring these kinds of benefits into our lives. Instead of waiting, we are creating new answers, more breaks, second chances.

Let me give you another living, breathing example. Her name is Patti Meese. She is the epitome of what I'm talking about. I call her the Energizer bunny of Parkinson's disease. She was diagnosed around seven years ago, or about three and a half years before my diagnosis. I sometimes tease that she is twice as old as I am in Parkinson's years. She tells me that if I want to live to see seven years, I should pipe down.

After her diagnosis, she quickly found herself struggling physically. Her posture became stooped, she was shuffling, and her left leg began to drag. In her words, she truly believed that she would have been in a wheelchair by now. So, what changed?

Well, she did. Instead of waiting to see if she might magically get better, she began to study as much as she could about Parkinson's. She believed knowledge was power. She discovered existing physical therapy programs such as LSVT BIG, NeuroFit PWR!Gym, water aerobics, and cycling. She saw the reversal of some of her physical symptoms and felt like she once again had her life back! To celebrate these accomplishments, she raised money for Parkinson's research by riding her bicycle in six-inch stilettos. I, of course, can think of much easier ways to raise money for research, but probably it wouldn't be nearly as entertaining.

Then, for a while, she lost her voice, and, as she described it, her joy, as well. She loved to sing, so she found a unique choral group for people with Parkinson's, their spouses and caregivers. The group was called ... wait for it, wait for it ... the Tremble Clefs! (Those of us with Parkinson's have nothing if not our sense of humor!) The songs and the music that the Tremble Clefs use are designed specifically to increase both the participants' vocal quality and volume. It is musical therapy for the vocal chords and the heart. To Patti's amazement, she got her voice back!

Now you see why I call her the Energizer bunny, but that's not all. To show the world that Parkinson's patients still have game (my words, not hers), she entered and was selected to be a contestant in the 2013 Ms. Senior Arizona Pageant. She walked away as First Runner-Up for the whole deal! I love that she won the talent portion of the contest by singing the song made famous in 1989 by Gloria Estefan, "Get On Your Feet." Do you remember the chorus? "Get on your feet, get up and make it happen! Get on your feet, stand up and take some action!" The verses talk about someone who is tired of trying, whose spirit is dying, but the answer is within; you just have to find it. Then the song returns to the inspiring chorus.

It's almost as if Gloria Estefan and Dr. Seuss were in cahoots regarding the message of not waiting around.

Let's get back to Patti. When she moved from Arizona to North Carolina a few years ago, you might think she would have decided it was time to sit back, take a break, and rest on her laurels. Actually, she hasn't slowed down a bit. She was recently appointed state director for the Parkinson's Action Network (PAN). PAN is the unified voice of the Parkinson's community advocating for better treatments and a cure, primarily through legislation that benefits all people with Parkinson's. Oh, and she also decided to bring the Tremble Clefs to North Carolina. I think it's her way of paying it forward.

I was recently kidding Patti about her appearance at the Move it! Walk to read the governor's proclamation. I thought she should do something out of the ordinary, like parachute in or hang glide to the center of the track. She said she would if I would, but we were just joking. At least, I hope she was joking. Of course, neither one of us had met Irene, yet. She would have done it in a heartbeat—as long as that handsome young fellow came along for the ride!

Chapter Two
Wiring

Do not conform to the pattern of this world, but be transformed by the renewing of your mind. —Romans 12:2

I now have electricity flowing through my brain. It's no big deal, other than the fact that I now have electricity flowing through my brain. But we all do. Much of our brain activity, nervous system functions, pain messaging, and so forth are driven by electric currents. However, I now have a state-of the-art neurostimulator that shoots somewhere between 130-160 pulses of juice per second directly into my brain. I also tend to turn on ceiling fans and open garage doors as I pass by.

I was selected as a candidate and then approved to be a recipient of what is known as deep brain stimulation (or DBS)—not to be confused with deep brain *simulation*, a mistake I made on my social media page the other day that made it sound like I was only pretending to have a brain. So, what does the stimulator do? It sends those constant pulses I mentioned and stimulates areas in your brain to help reduce the symptoms associated with Parkinson's, while also reducing the need for medications.

If you're completely unfamiliar with DBS and you're a science fiction fan, here's how my geek daughter explained my upcoming procedures to her friends and colleagues:

- Phase 1: The Frankenstein. They drill four screws into his skull. No big deal. They need them for mapping purposes.
- Phase 2: The Cyborg. This is when assimilation begins and they put the robotic parts [i.e. electrodes] into his brain.
- Phase 3: The Iron Man. This is when they put the battery pack in his chest to keep the robot brain running.
- Phase 4: The Terminator—specifically, *Rise of the Machines*. Before this step, all his robot parts will lay dormant. On this day, the good folks from Skynet will power him up and the machine will take over. Beware!

If you don't understand any of that, don't worry. I'll explain later in non-sci-fi terms. The main thing is that they do this in stages or phases. I think the time gaps are there to give the brain time to adjust to the new invasion of privacy at each interval—and I do mean *invasion*.

~

My choice of verse for this chapter is a little tongue in cheek. The author, Paul, is talking about the spiritual transformation of the mind, not the physical brain itself. Paul was in no way thinking about the insertion of a neurostimulator for a brain suffering from a dopamine deficiency. At least, I'm pretty sure that he wasn't, but I might be able to draw a parallel between what God wants to do in us spiritually and what my neurologist is hoping takes place in my actual, physical brain.

First, let's look at the context of this verse. Paul is writing a rather lengthy epistle to the Christian believers in Rome. Some say he wrote more than usual because he had not yet visited the capital city of the Roman Empire. He would make it there eventually, but that visit would not happen until after this letter was sent and received. This was Paul's attempt to catch them up on what everyone else was hearing—the teaching of an apostle concerning what it meant to be a Christian. If that's true, it seems they had a lot of catching up to do—sixteen chapters' worth!

In his opening greeting to these Christ-followers, you may notice something different. As was the custom in those days, the writer of an epistle first declared who was writing, instead of at the end as we are accustomed to nowadays. Thus, Romans begins: "Paul, a servant of Christ Jesus, called to be an apostle and set apart for the gospel of God" (Romans 1:1). Evidently, Paul couldn't resist starting on the teaching part of the epistle because for the next six verses he explains what he meant by "gospel of God." Paul tended to wax eloquent in his letters, which is a nice way of saying that he got a little long-winded.

But when we finally get to verse seven of chapter 1, after the explanation, Paul then makes it known to whom he directed this letter. "To all in Rome who are loved by God and called to be his holy people: Grace and peace to you from God our Father and from the Lord Jesus Christ" (Romans 1:7). It's that latter part of the first sentence that I want you to notice: "called to be his holy people." Literally, Paul says that the Romans believers were called to be the "saints" or the "holy ones" of God. Did Paul mean that they were to be "holy" like God is holy? Why, yes. Yes, he did. Then, he takes the sixteen chapters to explain how.

He doesn't start off very hopefully. In Romans 3, he tells these "saints" in Rome:

As it is written:

"There is no one righteous, not even one;
there is no one who understands;
there is no one who seeks God.
All have turned away,
they have together become worthless;
there is no one who does good,
not even one" (Romans 3:10-12).

It sounds encouraging, right? He nails the lid on the coffin with verse 23: "For all have sinned and fall short of the glory of God" (Romans 3:23).

This is terrible news, don't you think? But the good news, which is the literal meaning of the word *gospel*, follows in the very next verse: "And all are justified freely by his grace through the redemption that came by Christ Jesus" (Romans 3:24). Just as all have sinned, so all have been justified freely through what Jesus did on the cross. The only requirement is faith. What all this means is that God credited to us or declared us righteous and holy because of what Jesus did. But are we truly righteous and holy like God? Not by a long shot! I mean, have you met us? We who call ourselves Christians can be some of the most judgmental and grace-less people you've ever had the displeasure of knowing. One or two may be getting it right, but if you take those two out of the picture—perhaps Mother Teresa and Billy Graham—the pickings get slimmer. My apologies to those Christians who are trying to be less judgmental and more full of grace.

Surely, Paul would have been another exception, you might be thinking, *free from sin and temptation.* Well, listen to what he writes in Romans 7 and judge for yourself:

> I do not understand what I do. For what I want to do I do not do, but what I hate I do. ... For I know that good itself does not dwell in me, that is, in my sinful nature. For I have the desire to do what is good, but I cannot carry it out. For I do not do the good I want to do, but the evil I do not want to do—this I keep on doing (Romans 7:15, 18-19).

How can God still see us as holy and righteous, if most of us probably feel as if we're in the same boat as Paul? Because, if you will, God is looking through Jesus-colored glasses. It's corny, but true.

But does all that mean we will never change, never get better? No, it just means that we are a work in progress. Earlier, I mentioned Billy Graham who is very famous here in my hometown of Charlotte, North Carolina. His wife, Ruth, passed away several years ago, and she was buried on the grounds of the Billy Graham Library. You may not know the simple words she decided to have inscribed on her gravestone: "End of Construction. Thank you for your patience." I believe she understood what Paul was saying in Romans 7: "I am an imperfect sinner until the day I die, but God's goal for me is to transform me into the person he wants me to be."

Do you remember Romans 12:2? "Do not conform to the pattern of this world, but be transformed by the renewing of your mind." This is the transformation process that God wants to do in our hearts, spiritually speaking. Many Scriptures talk about this idea. Let me point to a few:

Being confident of this, that he who began a good work in you will carry it on to completion until the day of Christ Jesus (Philippians 1:6).

Not that I have already obtained all this, or have already arrived at my goal, but I press on to take hold of that for which Christ Jesus took hold of me. Brothers and sisters, I do not consider myself yet to have taken hold of it. But one thing I do: Forgetting what is behind and straining toward what is ahead, I press on toward the goal to win the prize for which God has called me heavenward in Christ Jesus (Philippians 3:12-14).

Dear friends, now we are children of God, and what we will be has not yet been made known. But we know that when Christ appears, we shall be like him, for we shall see him as he is (1 John 3:2).

And from the same letter to the Romans, Paul in chapter 8 writes: "For those God foreknew he also predestined to be conformed to the image of his Son, that he might be the firstborn among many brothers and sisters" (Romans 8:29). The Message paraphrase of the Bible puts it this way: "God knew what he was doing from the very beginning. He decided from the outset to shape the lives of those who love him along the same lines as the life of his Son."

If you're missing it, here's what we are saying: We're all in process—under construction—slowly being transformed into the kind of life that Jesus lived. We are not all becoming messiahs. There's a term for that particular mental condition. But we are all trying to learn to love like Jesus loved, extend grace like he extended grace, speak truth like he spoke truth, and so on. It's a lifelong process. No one will reach perfection before they die. But you probably already knew that, right?

In his book *Mere Christianity*, C.S. Lewis explains what a thorough job God does when he transforms a life that is submitted to him. It's like we're a house and we invite God to come in and do a little remodeling and a few minor repairs. God does not stop there, however. He adds a new story and a few extra bedrooms, maybe a tower or two and beautiful courtyards. We were just wanting a better home, but he is making something nice enough for him to live in.

So, how do we submit ourselves to this transformation process? That is, how exactly do we let God transform us? I am oversimplifying here, but it really boils down to living in tune with God's words and his Spirit. How is our mind renewed or reprogrammed so that we live more as Jesus did? By getting in sync with the things that he taught and with the way that he lived. You could say that we learn to march to the beat of a different drummer—Jesus himself. His rhythm marks our step. His beat guides our thinking. His song becomes the theme music to the movie of our lives. OK, are you ready for the parallel now?

~

The other day, I ran across a video on the National Parkinson Foundation website. I was interested in the answer to one particular question: How does the DBS device work? The man in the video was Dr. Michael S. Okun, author of the current top-selling book on Parkinson's as of this writing, *Parkinson's Treatment: 10*

Secrets to a Happier Life. Here was his exact answer to my question:

> We actually don't know the answer to that question. It turns out that we put these tiny little electrodes into brain regions, and we introduce essentially white noise. We can change the noise we introduce by making the pulses longer or shorter. We can give them at faster or slower frequencies. We can turn up the volume or the voltage of these devices. We get varying side effects and benefits when we do this. When we stimulate in different regions of the brain, we get different benefits and different side effects.

That was his answer. A little worrisome, don't you think? But then he explains further:

> Now, how does it actually work? Well, when we turn these devices on, it makes a little field, almost like a sphere—like a globe—a field of electricity comes out of the tip of one or more of these electrodes, and it affects several of the different cells, it affects the chemicals, it affects everything that is within that sphere. We believe that we're changing the conversations between different brain regions. If we take those little tiny microelectrodes, the tip of which is about the size of a hair, we crawl down and we listen to those cells singing, they're singing songs. By introducing electricity into the brain, into this globe, into this sphere area, we can change the song that they sing. The songs that they sing are very important to the absolute function, to the outcome for patients. We believe that in some eloquent way, we're altering these brain conversations ... . By changing the abnormal

conversation, we seem to be improving the symptoms of patients."

Changing the songs that the brain cells sing? Altering the brain conversations? Doesn't that sound a whole lot like marching to the beat of a different drummer? The new rhythm marks our step. The new beat guides our thinking. The new song becomes the theme music to the movie of our lives. Now, do you see why I thought this verse might just work?

~

Phase 1 was a joke waiting to happen. After all, they were drilling four screws into my skull. I heard every possible version of, "So, do you, or did you, have a loose screw?" during the days immediately before and following the procedure.

Five people were in the room for that procedure: my wife—only because she is not squeamish whatsoever; the representative (who also has become a good friend) from Medtronic, the maker of the neurostimulator; the neurosurgeon, whom I liked from the first time I met him; and the neurosurgeon's nurse, a very nice young lady who made sure I was doing OK at all times. Oh, and I was there, too.

The first step was to inject local anesthesia at the four entry points. The doctor said it would feel like a bee sting. Luckily, as a kid I had been stung in the head by a bee. (Go back and read that last sentence, and tell me if you ever would have thought about putting together those particular words before.) It's the one vivid memory I have from when I was three years old. I was following my grandfather's footsteps as he tilled his garden for planting. Papaw drove the tiller right past the beehives that my father kept. He walked by the bees without incident, but as I followed his path, they were a little less accommodating. The first one stung me on the top of my head. I ran screaming toward the house, yelling, "Dot me!" which, being translated, means: "He got me!" The second bee came low and hard, and I yelled: "Dot me, again!" I'm not sure how many bees found my head that day, but the two phrases I yelled became some of those kids-say-the-darndest-things sayings that we repeated over and over as a family.

All that to tell you, I knew what was coming that day, and as the doctor circled my head injecting bee-like stings in four different areas, I relayed that story and said, "Dot me!" and "Dot me again!" right on cue. Then I heard the drill. I didn't have any cute stories about drills.

The doctor then told us a story about wasps from his childhood, and I can almost swear he was using both hands to describe the event to the other three people in the room. I remember thinking, *Both hands on the drill, Doc!* Of course, he kept them there at all times, and all four screws went in without incident.

My wife asked if I could hear the drill in my ear and inside my head. I told her I could hear it everywhere. Twenty minutes later, however, we were done. I went in for a CT scan to confirm that the screws were in the right places. They were, and it's a good thing. I did not want to return to the drill room and reverse those screws out and rethread them in new places. Once I had passed that test, I was soon sent home with pain meds and a turban of white gauze. For days, I told everyone I had a splitting headache, literally.

This first phase was called the fiducial placement. *Fiducial* means "a fixed point of reference." It's my understanding that these fiducial screws were used for mapping the best placement of the electrodes, which would take place in Phase 2. We were eight days away from the big surgery. That seemed like an eternity. I tried to fill the time with visits from friends, writing this book as my brain allowed, and even going a few towns away for a book signing. Nothing could take away the low-grade anxiety in the back of my mind. The success rate was in the mid-90s, and the other possibilities were extremely low, but they were there, with all the baggage that came with each result:

1. The surgery would not work and the neurostimulator would have to be removed.
2. The surgery would cause permanent brain damage.
3. The surgery could cause death.

Isn't it funny how we fixate on the low probabilities instead of that big, old success rate? I was a pain to live with that week before. No, actually, I was a pain that whole month before! I gave lots of just-in-case talks and have-I-said-it-often-enough? speeches. My family and closest friends were probably worn out from all the honesty.

A little later, I realized something about fiducial placement. The root word is the same as that of *trust* and *faith*. A person can be said to have a fiducial dependence on God. Eventually, I can say I got there, and I owe most of that to the ones who kept pushing me in that direction. One of my former high school students at the Christian academy where I taught called me and prayed with me the night before. His prayer was straight to the point, "God. I know you're not done with Mr. Woodall, because he's not done helping me sort out my life." Whoever taught that young man his Bible classes must have been one heck of a teacher!

Phase 2 dawned bright and early the next day. Well, it

was early at least; it was still dark when we drove down to the hospital. My wife and daughters were there; my parents; Cheryl's mom; my pastor; and some wonderful friends, one of whom had already had the DBS surgery and was there as living proof of the mid-90s success figure. I didn't hear about all of them until much later. On my side of the hospital was a smaller group: the neurosurgeon, his P.A., my neurologist, my friend from Medtronic, and a handful of other voices that I did not recognize. I saw them all when I first entered the operating room and a little while later when I woke up during surgery! Yes, you read that right, during surgery!

In the middle of the procedure, when it was time to insert the electrodes, they woke me, and I remember almost every second of it. Well, I think I do. Cheryl and I had listened to a comedian on the way to the hospital that morning, so the first thing I remember saying was, "Do you guys want to hear a joke?"

Evidently, that is not the question people ask when they first wake up, so they told me to hold that thought for a few minutes. Then, they said, "Fire away!" So, I told them one of the jokes I had heard that morning, from Jim Gaffigan, who lives in New York City.

"What is the difference between a New York public restroom and a New York crime scene?" The punch line is, "At least they'll clean up after a crime scene." Hey, I didn't say it was a great joke.

Well, that set the mood, and that part of the brain surgery was a whole lot of … fun. That may seem far-fetched, but it was. I was cracking jokes, and everyone began to fire them right back. There was a fair amount of laughter, which was good for me.

They probably kept me awake a tad too long, because I ended up offending my neurologist, who is a highly intelligent woman; distinguished in her field; respected by her colleagues and co-workers; has a beautiful smile and a wonderful bedside manner; and who, I hope, reads books written by patients still trying to apologize in any and every way possible.

At one point, she noticed that my left arm was less flexible than my right, and she asked me about it. I told her that my right arm was the more athletic one. "Give me a baseball in my right hand, and I can throw straight and fast," I explained. "Put it in my left hand, and I throw like a girl."

Dead silence.

"Oh, do you now?" she said, quietly.

"I mean, I throw like a wimpy, wimpy boy," I stuttered quickly, but she wasn't buying it. I tried to formally apologize later, but it was to no avail.

With a smirk, she explained "If you think I'm going to let you off that easily, you don't know me very well."

One of my daughters came up with an idea. I ended up buying the neurologist's soon-to-be-born baby daughter a small, pink baseball glove and a Velcro-sticking ball a few weeks later. I delivered it to her office with a note that read: "To the best pitcher, catcher, and hitter that baseball has ever seen." She later confirmed that I was slowly but surely digging myself out of the hole.

Another thing I remember about being awake during that procedure was the adjustments she made to the neurostimulator at one point. She asked me to look at her and tell her if she was in focus. I told her I could see two of her, standing side by side. She tweaked the settings and asked again. I still saw two of her, but now they were one on top of the other. She tweaked again, and my vision corrected. The whole process was amazing. She was fine-tuning the songs that the brain cells would sing.

I spent the night in ICU, and again the splitting headache was the worst part of that experience. It took several attempts at pain medication to bring that under control, but we finally conquered the worst of it. I may have been guessing low on my pain level. They always ask the question: "What is your pain level on a scale from one to ten?"

"Well, what's a ten?" I asked.

"Being run over by a train," they answered. I had this sneaky suspicion that my pain was no way near that category, so I said a seven or eight. Next time I have brain surgery, though, I'm going to say ten until it stops hurting.

Phase 3 was another quickie. About a week later, I went in to have the battery pack installed. They didn't wake me up for this one. Maybe they thought I might make another bad joke or offend someone. They marked which side I preferred with a marker and installed the pack not so far under the skin. It felt like a deck of cards just inside my chest. The electrode wires now ran from my brain to my battery pack. I went home the same day. I like to think I have one rock-solid ab, about twelve inches too high. All the DBS parts were in place at this point. Now I just needed someone to turn me on. As you can imagine, Phase 4 brought its own share of expected jokes.

For Phase 4, I went back to my neurologist's office. She inspected the surgery sites, pronounced them as healing properly, and then began to explain the apparatus she held in her hands. It was the switch that was about to be flipped. I was a little nervous. I had no idea what to expect. Can you feel electricity when it flows into your brain? The answer turned out to be: Yes. And no. It depends on the voltage.

She began at the lowest level, and we gradually worked up to the highest that I could tolerate without showing significant physical reaction. At the lowest settings, I first felt nothing, then some tingling along my arm, and a muscle that seemed to twitch involuntarily. As the voltage increased, so did my body's responses. I felt some dizziness and a pull on my facial muscles that caused me to turn and lean toward the side she was working on. At the highest level, it felt like my tongue was hanging out of my head and my eyes were rolling around involuntarily. There was no pain, mind you, and between every adjustment, my neurologist was checking my flexibility, coordination, and walking ability. She took extensive notes all the time.

When I arrived at the office that day, I had taken no medications since the night before. By the time we were done, I was walking down the hallway and back without a shuffle. The next few visits continued the tweaking process, gradually increasing voltage and lessening my dependence on the meds. The neurostimulator performed as advertised. It gave me my best day on meds without having to take all my meds.

Or, as I like to say, it began to sing new songs to my brain, and it changed the conversations that my brain cells were having with each other. I like the sound of that.

Chapter Three
Weeping

Jesus wept. —John 11:35

Several years ago, I went to my first educational symposium on Parkinson's. A local hospital hosted the event. During the meet and greet time, we were shaking hands all around and I met an elderly man with Parkinson's. He was there with his son. I remember that the man had fairly pronounced dyskinesia—those jerky movements that sometimes roll like waves through one's body—but that was not the symptom that shook me to my core. What I vividly remember was that he cried the whole time I was speaking with him. Normally, I don't have that effect on people. Usually I can either make them laugh or, worst-case scenario, put them to sleep, but this guy wept in response to everything I said. I turned to his son for support, and he quietly said, "He cries about everything now." I hadn't heard of this symptom yet.

When I told my movement disorder specialist about it, he immediately had a term: *emotional incontinence*. Cute, right? Emotional incontinence is when a person laughs or cries uncontrollably and involuntarily. Really? I jokingly asked if they made a Depends for that. But my real question was: Does every symptom associated with Parkinson's have to be a socially awkward behavior? I mean, can't we catch a break here?

I think I may have a slightly less-pronounced version of this symptom. I do seem to cry and/or laugh much more often than I used to and with much more intensity.

Cheryl agrees with that assessment: "You do lose it more frequently." I have written elsewhere that, on quite a few occasions, my daughters have brought me to the point of such uncontrollable, red-faced episodes of laughter that I have actually had to beg them to stop for a minute so I could breathe again.

On the other end of the spectrum, sometimes all it takes is a good book or a movie to move me to tears. I may have always had that tendency. I just seem to get there much more easily than in previous years. A prime example is *Saving Private Ryan*, a Steven Spielberg movie starring Tom Hanks and Matt Damon. Tom Hanks plays Captain Miller. Miller and his squad of soldiers are sent out to find Private Ryan (played by Matt Damon), the only surviving brother of four who went off to war together. Their assignment is to find Ryan and send him home to his mourning mother. Well—spoiler alert—all but two of the soldiers on this mission are killed.

The part that always gets me is when Captain Miller whispers his last words to Ryan. He pulls him close and says through his clenched teeth: "Earn this … earn it!"

The movie fast forwards to an elderly Ryan, nearing the end of his life and standing at Miller's grave. He chokes out the words: "Every day I think about what you said to me that day on the bridge. I tried to live my life the best that I could. I hope that was enough. I hope that, at least in

your eyes, I've earned what all of you have done for me."
His wife comes up to see if he's OK, and he desperately
pleads with her: "Tell me I've lived a good life. Tell me I'm
a good man."

I get misty-eyed just typing it.

The good news is that I haven't completely folded and
started watching Hallmark movies, thank goodness, but
don't even mention *Band of Brothers*, another
Spielberg/Hanks collaboration. If Cheryl walks in and that
mini-series is on, she tosses in a box or two of tissues and
quietly slips away.

I always respond, "I'm not crying this time."

She says: "I know, honey. I know."

The problem is that I don't know if this is all
connected with my Parkinson's, or just a sign that I'm
getting older and more sentimental. My girls think it's the
latter. However, since I discovered the term, I like to blame
it on the Parkinson's as often as I can. It's come in handy
over the last few years.

~

Sadly, last year my father-in-law passed away. *Sadly*
does not seem like a big enough word to express the depth
and range of emotions we experienced. Cheryl's family
asked me to say a few words at the funeral. It was a disaster
waiting to happen. I was followed by two of the nephews.
One was a colonel in the army, a former paratrooper turned
JAG officer. He's a no-nonsense, just-the-facts kind of
man's man. The second was an immigration agent, a
barrel-chested, motorcycle-riding tough guy, who once
punched a shark in the face to rescue his son. My father-in-
law's brother went next, a six-foot-four, broad-shouldered,

successful businessman who spoke with a deep, booming, authoritative voice.

When I stepped onto the platform, I talked about the first time I met my future father-in-law. He was standing at the door of his house in Eagle Pass, Texas, holding a shotgun in his hand. I had driven his daughter all the way home from college in central Florida.

His first words to me were: "Let me just finish cleaning this. Then we can talk for a minute." Then he grinned and said, "Just kidding. Come on in!"

Cheryl just beamed at me the whole time, as if to say, "Isn't he just the best?" I told the crowd that I realized at that moment that I was marrying a daddy's girl.

I spoke for a few more minutes about his love for his family—how much he cherished his lovely wife, his two beautiful daughters, his four gorgeous granddaughters, and the newly arrived great grandson—and his love for God. Where I began to lose it, however, was when I commented about the two great examples of husbands and fathers that God had given me: first, my own father, who was sitting in the room that day to pay his respects, and then my father-in-law. Both had recently celebrated their fiftieth wedding anniversaries, and both were adored by all of their now-grown children. I explained that it was as if God were somehow hedging his bets with me to make sure he got through this thick-skinned, hard head of mine—to make sure I got it right.

I never lost it completely, but my voice cracked several times, and at a few points I had to resort to Lamaze-type breathing to hold it together. I felt like an overly sensitive, weepy mess when I finally sat down. My sister-in-law told me later that she would have been hurt if I had not broken down.

It made me feel a little better when the three men who followed me all did the same thing, matter-of-fact starts with tearful finishes. I went to each of them after the service and said, "You know, one of the symptoms of Parkinson's is emotional incontinence. That's my excuse for what just happened. So, what's yours?" Then I quickly slipped away. After all, they were bigger than me.

~

In most of my talks to support groups, I encourage listeners to focus on the positive, opt for optimism, maintain a good attitude, and so forth. I believe all those practices are important if we want to live well with our diagnosis. But times for grief and mourning do come. Solomon wrote a simple, yet profound, poem in Ecclesiastes 3:

> There is a time for everything,
> and a season for every activity under the heavens:
> a time to be born and a time to die,
> a time to plant and a time to uproot,
> a time to kill and a time to heal,
> a time to tear down and a time to build,
> *a time to weep* and a time to laugh,
> *a time to mourn* and a time to dance,
> a time to scatter stones and a time to gather them,
> a time to embrace and a time to refrain from embracing,
> a time to search and a time to give up,
> a time to keep and a time to throw away,
> a time to tear and a time to mend,
> a time to be silent and a time to speak,
> a time to love and a time to hate,

a time for war and a time for peace
(Ecclesiastes 3:1-8, italics mine).

My advice to support groups remains the same, but
there are seasons in our lives when we must acknowledge
and face the sadness we feel. We must let ourselves go
through the process of dealing with the pain of loss. That's
what grief is, a process.

All who spoke at my father-in-law's funeral had
experienced a significant loss. We were working through
the grief, each in his own way. Most of us with any time on
the planet know what that feels like. Anyone who has
suffered through the death of someone dear recognizes the
hurt, the heartbreak, and the healing that has to take place.
And when I say *healing*, that may merely mean that
eventually the emotions become less raw and nothing more.
Still, it takes time for even that to happen.

But there is another kind of grief, although the process
remains the same. We who have been diagnosed with a
chronic disease also experience a profound sense of loss—
the loss of our health, independence, and mobility, among
other things. We mourn because the life we once knew is
no longer our reality and we now must be dependent on
numerous variables, such as our medications, the kindness
and the schedules of others, and our own much-more-
limited abilities. I've already seen it in my life.

Up until my diagnosis, the task of driving anywhere
was mine. I walked to the driver's side of the car almost
without thinking. Cheryl always went to the passenger side.
If the trip was long, then Cheryl may have helped do some
of the driving a little farther down the highway, but I
always took the first shift. Now, nothing is automatic. Who
drives depends on how my meds are working or perceived
to be working. Now, as often as not, Cheryl says, "I'm

driving." This change in our lives may seem trivial to some, but I saw it as a shift in the tectonic plates of our thirty-plus-year relationship. During the lengthy waiting periods of my DBS phases, I faced a complete ban on driving. I was miserable those two or three weeks. I was completely at the mercy of others, and the loss of privilege was almost unbearable. I couldn't even contemplate the very real possibility that this ban might one day be my permanent situation.

I refer to the kind of grief that I've been describing as *living grief.* The term is not mine, nor is it new. It is often used to describe the emotions of those, for instance, whose loved one has developed dementia. Although the patient is still very much alive, their mental state has left them a different person, a person with limited memory of the past and sometimes no recognition whatsoever of the person who just walked in the room—even though the "visitor" is the spouse, son, or daughter of the patient. The one with dementia is already gone, if not physically, then in most other ways.

In the case of the person with Parkinson's, both the patient and the caregiver can suffer this kind of grief. They are mourning not the physical death of a person, but the loss of who that person once was, the abilities that he or she once had, the freedom that he or she once enjoyed, the hopes that he or she once held. The loss is just as real as the actual loss of a loved one.

In the support group that I lead with my buddy Vince, we took a survey of what kind of physical symptoms or limitations—losses, if you will—we were now experiencing. Our group ranges in age from fifty-two to eighty-two years, with diagnoses from three to thirteen years out. In the parenthetical side notes, we tried to make the list humorous, but there was no getting around the sense that our lives had been drastically affected by this thing called Parkinson's:

- Shuffling gait (But at least we can keep up with our toddler grandchildren.)
- Freezing (It's not because the A/C is cranking the temperature too low, but because our legs won't move.)
- Tremor (It can be just the legs or hands or the whole body, on one or both sides—versatile!)
- Rigidity (Our arms don't swing or move when we walk; it's excellent for river dancing, however.)
- Drooling (It's especially when pretty girls go by; it may not be associated with PD!)
- Difficulty with handwriting (It's too sloppy or too small to see—a matter of perspective really.)
- Talking too softly or muttering (But the truth is, some comments are better left unheard.)
- Losing sense of smell and taste (This works to our advantage on many occasions.)
- Drifting to one side or the other when walking or sitting (And, often, when voting.)
- Hesitancy with words and thoughts (Again, this may or may not be associated with PD.)
- Memory problems (It helps to write a list, if we can only remember where we left the list.)
- Sleep apnea (Is it PD-related or weight-related? Some insisted this was better left unanswered.)
- Active, nonsensical hallucinations and dreams (Is it PD or the pizza we ate before bed?)
- Split or double vision (What helps? Prism on glasses, covering one eye, or a permanent wink.)
- Spatial coordination (We might miss the chair when we sit down, and then pretend we meant to.)

- Eating difficulties (This is primarily with tremor, especially with foods like green peas.)
- Lipstick application problems (This only affected certain group members. We're not saying whom.)
- Dystonia (It's the curling of hands and/or feet. Stretch exercises help as does switching hands to write.)
- Imbalance (We have a real fear of falling. It's one of the most repeated symptoms of our group.)
- Constipation (No details, please.)

All of these very specific symptoms or physical limitations can easily be grouped into loss categories: mobility, control, bodily function, the life we once knew. On the day we made the symptoms list, in an attempt to end the meeting on a high note, we also made a list of the things we could still do. That is always my policy in group meetings: We send people on their way with a bit of hope. You know, as in: Shuffle on! However, since the theme of this chapter has to do with grief and mourning, let's linger on the negative for just a few more pages, specifically on the question: What is this grief process that we must go through?

~

In her 1969 book, *On Death and Dying*, Elizabeth Kübler-Ross contended that there were five stages in the grief process: denial, anger, bargaining, depression, and acceptance. Of course, not everyone experiences all five of these stages, or if one does, one doesn't go through each stage with the same intensity. The order of the stages is not set in concrete, either. My own journey through living grief has touched on four of the five thus far.

I think everyone experiences denial. I call it the "shock absorber of grief." The loss is felt so acutely that our minds need time to adjust to the reality of the situation. It's more like disbelief that this can really be happening in our lives. We've all seen a movie scene where a wife receives the news that her husband has been killed on the battlefield or in the line of duty and she collapses in a heap, screaming: "No, no, no. It not's true. It can't be true!" Denial gives our hearts and minds some needed space between the way things were and the ways things are. It usually is short-lived because the cold, hard, objective truth eventually comes in and kicks it out, but temporary denial keeps us sane. I'm convinced of that.

The bargaining stage is the one that I haven't really experienced yet. It's in this stage that an individual tries to make some kind of cosmic deal with God, or the universe, or whoever or whatever his or her Higher Power might be. The person might make some kind of promise: "God, if you heal me, I'll serve you as a missionary, or I'll be a pastor, or I'll feed the poor, or I'll do all three." Maybe that's why I don't feel like I've been through this one, yet. On all the above promises, I've been there, done that, got the T-shirt. Maybe my bargaining stage will look different.

I know the remaining three stages well: anger, depression, and eventually acceptance. When it comes to my Parkinson's, I camped out in the first two for weeks, maybe months, but I believe I have reached acceptance. It's a reluctant acceptance, mind you, with occasional peeks out the door to see if a miracle or a cure might be coming down the road. In other words, I've gotten to acceptance because it's the only place to go. If denial is the shock absorber, acceptance is the cruise control that keeps me moving toward sanity, normality, and functionality.

I recently spoke with a pastor friend who also has a chronic disease and is going through some of the same experiences I am. He asked me to speak at his church on some of the themes from my first book and, specifically, on the idea of God saying *no* to our requests for healing. Afterward, we talked about the anger he was feeling, including anger toward God. I told him that such feelings were normal, a familiar part of grief that nearly everyone experiences when he or she suffers a loss.

I have found that anger will sooner or later transition to depression, mainly because we come to the conclusion that our diatribes do not change anything, no matter how much we yell and scream. And depression eventually gives way to acceptance, primarily because we realize that our sadness likewise changes nothing. Or sometimes depression comes first, then anger. The order is not important. Ultimately, we have to *accept* that acceptance is the only possible outcome. I guess it's possible to never get to that place, but who would want to live like that?

I realize that I'm making the grief process and the five stages sound much too orderly. Every psychologist, counselor, and pastor is screaming, "It's not that simple!" I wholeheartedly agree. Much like with Parkinson's, the road may be different for everyone, and few of those roads are perfectly sequenced with all five stages from some textbook. Whenever human emotions are involved, everything is much more complicated. But I'll bet you already knew that.

While I mentioned earlier that I occasionally peek out of the acceptance stage to see if a miracle or a cure has materialized, I also have been known to let anger and depression slip back into my heart and mind. That is, I feel the need to step back out to vent ... or to cry. The former is understandable. The latter? That's probably just that emotional incontinence thing again.

~

So, where is God in all this? What part does he play in the grieving process? Those questions lead me back to the opening verse for this chapter: "Jesus wept" (John 11:35). Those two words speak volumes. When you understand the reason why Jesus wept, it's quite an overwhelming thought to consider. Let me set up the story for you.

John 11 begins with the news that a man named Lazarus was sick. Lazarus and his two sisters, Martha and Mary, were close friends of Jesus. Lazarus is described as the one Jesus loved. Mary is the woman who poured perfume on Jesus' feet and then wiped and dried them with her hair. The women send word to Jesus of Lazarus' sickness, no doubt expecting him to come immediately.

When Jesus gets the news, he makes a strange comment: "This sickness will not end in death" (John 11:4). And then he decides to stay where he is two more days. He's in no hurry, it seems, to get to Lazarus's house and come to the aid of his friend. I mean, the reason that Martha and Mary sent for Jesus in the first place undoubtedly is because they wanted Jesus to work a miracle. But he doesn't come and Lazarus dies. Jesus' prediction seemingly proves untrue.

Then Jesus announces: "Our friend Lazarus has fallen asleep; but I am going there to wake him up" (John 11:4).

The disciples misunderstand and reply: "Lord, if he sleeps, he will get better" (John 11:12). They think Jesus is referring to actual sleeping and that with the proper rest Lazarus will be able to recuperate from whatever illness has sickened him.

So, now Jesus tells them what he actually meant: "Lazarus is dead." Then he adds: "And for your sake I am glad I was not there, so that you may believe" (John 11:14-15).

I'm quite sure they have no idea what he's talking about. One thing's for sure: They are about to be utterly shocked.

When Jesus and company finally arrive in Bethany, they discover that Lazarus has already been in the tomb for four days. So much for the sickness not ending in death! Immediately upon hearing that Jesus is coming, Martha runs out to meet him.

She minces no words: "Lord, if you had been here, my brother would not have died" (John 11:21).

Jesus says to her, "Your brother will rise again" (John 11:23). He's hinting at something here, but she doesn't catch it.

Martha answers, "I know he will rise again in the resurrection at the last day" (John 11:24). She's thinking of some point in the future.

Jesus hints again, "I am the resurrection and the life. The one who believes in me will live, even though they die" (John 11:25).

She's still not comprehending what's about to happen. Who could? Then she runs inside her house and finds Mary. "He's asking for you," she says. I've often wondered why she says that. There's no mention in the narrative of Jesus asking for Mary. Could it be that the strange conversation between Martha and Jesus prompts her to send her sister out? Maybe Mary will be able to understand what he's trying to say.

So, Mary runs out to where Jesus is standing, and it's obvious that she and Martha have been discussing things because she begins with the very same question as her sister: "Lord, if you had been here, my brother would not have died" (John 11:32).

The next part of the narrative is enlightening. John writes:

> When Jesus saw her weeping, and the Jews who had come along with her also weeping, he was deeply moved in spirit and troubled. "Where have you laid him?" he asked. "Come and see, Lord;" they replied. *Jesus wept.* Then the Jews said, "See how he loved him!" (John 11:33-36, italics mine).

Why is Jesus weeping? The Jews standing nearby conclude it's because he loves Lazarus so much. Is Jesus sad because his friend has died? Is he sad that he had not arrived in time? I don't think it was either one.

He seems to have delayed his arrival on purpose, with a plan already in mind. And surely he already knows what he is going to do after he gets there. There are hints all through the narrative of the miracle to come. Jesus is about to raise a four-days-dead man from the grave. It's practice, you could say. Very soon he will have to do a similar miracle for a three-days-dead guy.

No, the explanation seems to be much simpler. I think he merely is touched by the sight of Martha and Mary weeping and all who are with them. The writer of the passage says that Jesus is deeply moved in his spirit, even troubled, at the sight of those who are mourning. The God-became-human Jesus is overwhelmed with the sadness his delay has caused. I believe he weeps out of empathy for those he loves. The sight of his dear friends crying moves him to tears, and he doesn't even struggle with emotional incontinence!

A verse in Hebrews compares Jesus with the high priests of the Old Testament and urges us to come to him with confidence. It then explains why: "For we do not have a high priest who is unable to empathize with our weaknesses, but we have one who has been tempted in every way, just as we are—yet he did not sin" (Hebrews 4:15).

In Philippians 2:7, Paul talks about the God-became-human transformation, explaining that Jesus "made himself nothing by taking the very nature of a servant, being made in human likeness." Jesus can empathize with us because he was one of us—human, complete with flesh and blood and all the same feelings and emotions that come with the package. He knows what sadness and pain feel like because he experienced them, too, along with every other kind of human emotion.

In another chapter, we'll talk about the existence of pain and suffering in the world and the ever-elusive answer to the *why* question. But for now, I believe we can say that in the midst of our suffering, God understands what we are going through, right down to the tears we shed. He weeps when we weep. He is saddened by what saddens us, the grief that we bear, and the pain that we suffer. And if all this is really true, then it means we have a God who genuinely cares for us. There might even be a verse or two in the Bible that says those very words. Check out 1 Peter 5:7, for an example.

The happy ending to the Lazarus story is that Jesus did raise his friend from the dead. I'm just guessing here, but I'm betting that there was even more crying that day, crying of a slightly different variety. Those tears probably did not fall until after the initial shock wore off, of course. Everyone stood there, undoubtedly, with mouths agape as Lazarus shuffled out of the tomb, still wrapped like a mummy, with linen strips from head to toe. In fact, Jesus had to prompt them, "Uh, you guys can take the grave clothes off now."

And if the Lazarus story is not enough, Luke records yet another funeral that Jesus attended, one where he raised yet another guy from the dead. This story does not say how-many-days-dead the young man happened to be. Neither does it say that Jesus wept, but he might have. But it does tell us what he felt when he saw the mourning mother: "When the Lord saw her, his heart went out to her and he said, 'Don't cry'" (Luke 7:13). That phrase "his heart went out" in our English translations is a single word in the original Greek, and it's only used twelve times in the New Testament. Every time, the word either refers to how Jesus felt in different sets of circumstances (e.g., seeing the multitudes that had not eaten for days, talking with the blind man and the leper who wanted to be healed), or Jesus uses the word to describe how someone else felt (e.g., the good Samaritan, the father of the prodigal son, and so on).

The literal meaning of this Greek word is "to experience something so deeply that your bowels move." I'm not kidding. In those days, the people believed that the bowels were the center of one's being, much like we say, "That broke my heart," and believe that the heart is the center of our emotions and feelings. But I digress. The point is that this very unusual word is only used by Jesus or used to refer to him. It means that when people were suffering or going through times of grief and distress, Jesus was touched in the very core of his being.

Other verses from the Bible seem to confirm that God is actively present in the midst of those times. Psalm 10:17 says: "You, Lord, hear the desire of the afflicted; you encourage them, and you listen to their cry." Psalm 22:24 assures: "For he has not despised or scorned the suffering of the afflicted one; he has not hidden his face from him but has listened to his cry for help." Perhaps my favorite is found in Psalm 23:4: "Even though I walk through the darkest valley [more famously known as the valley of the shadow of death], I will fear no evil, for you are with me; your rod and your staff, they comfort me."

The truth is that, while we must admit that we don't always understand the reasons God allows our suffering in the first place, we often come to realize that we tend to feel closest to God during the worst of that very suffering—his presence seems nearer, his voice seems clearer, that sort of thing.

Singer and songwriter Jeremy Camp, who lost his first wife to ovarian cancer, wrote a beautifully honest song to God shortly after her death. "I Still Believe" became one of his greatest hits. Google the lyrics when you get the opportunity.

It's all about still trusting and believing in God even though we don't understand the circumstances in which we find ourselves. The part that grabs my attention is that, in the middle of Jeremy's worst suffering, God was there, his grace falling like a gentle rain, actually washing away the pain.

You see, I believe that's exactly where God is during the grieving process—right in the thick of things, right beside us, right with us. Paul writes in 2 Corinthians these words: "Praise be to the God and Father of our Lord Jesus Christ, the Father of compassion and the God of all comfort, who comforts us in all our troubles, so that we can comfort those in any trouble with the comfort we ourselves receive from God" (2 Corinthians 1:3-4). I love that phrase: "The God of all comfort." It's comforting, don't you think?

Chapter Four
Why-ing Part 1

Why have you made me your target? Have I become a burden to you? —Job 7:20

Philip Yancey calls *why* "the question that never goes away." He wrote a book by that same title as a sequel to his first book on the subject, *Where is God When it Hurts?* I guess the first title was technically a *where* question, but it dealt with the *why* dilemma, as in: Why do bad things happen to good people? This paragraph is starting to sound dangerously close to the old Abbott and Costello "Who's On First?" comedy routine, so I'd better move on.

First, let me say that unless you're a theist—that is, someone who believes in God or allows for the possibility of a god or gods—this chapter is not for you. If you consider yourself to be a bona fide, tried and true, even-if-I-were-in-a-foxhole nontheist, then the following pages will deal with a moot point for you. That's because the *why* question assumes that there is someone or something out there controlling everything, and it, he, or she must give an answer for the evil and suffering in the world. If you are convinced that there cannot be, must not be, has never been, nor ever will be any kind of supernatural force, personal or otherwise, then feel free to skip this chapter. This one might be a tad heavy on the theologizing. After all, we're the ones with the problem—those of us who do believe in God and the Bible. We're the ones who must struggle with the fact that God does not always behave as we would like him to behave. And, boy, do we struggle.

Of course, I am extremely familiar with the argument that many nontheists point to as proof that God does not exist. It goes something like this: If God exists and he truly is all-powerful, then he could just wipe out evil, pain, and suffering in one fell swoop. And if he truly is all-loving, he would want to do that very thing on behalf of those that he loves. Thus, because we still have evil, pain, and suffering in abundance, then that should prove to the whole world that God does not exist.

Bart Ehrman has devoted his life to challenging the claims of Christianity. He's an award-winning and widely known professor at the University of North Carolina at Chapel Hill, and for many years he was the Chair of the Department of Religious Studies. His book titles tell the tale: *Misquoting Jesus: The Story Behind Who Changed the Bible and Why*; *Jesus, Interrupted: Revealing the Hidden Contradictions in the Bible (and Why We Don't Know About Them)*; *Forged: Writing in the Name of God—Why the Bible's Authors Are Not Who We Think They Are*; and *Forgery and Counterforgery: The Use of Literary Deceit in Early Christian Polemics.* Are you starting to get the picture that he might be on a mission?

One of his most popular books is titled, *God's Problem: How the Bible Fails to Answer Our Most Important Question—Why We Suffer.* In the opening pages of the book, Ehrman points to this one issue as the source of everything for him and relates that the problem of suffering has "haunted" him throughout his life. It's what led him to God when he was a youth and what led him to deny God's existence as he grew older.

I do not plan on debating Bart Ehrman any time soon. In fact, I tell high school students who go to UNC Chapel Hill that if they plan to take one of his courses, they should not try to out-argue him or convert him with their amazing logic and debate skills. He knows his stuff and probably is in the habit of eating underclassmen for breakfast. I don't know that for sure, but I would suspect that it's close to the truth.

However, I will argue that the title of his book, *God's Problem*, is a little misleading. The Bible does not fail to answer the question of why we suffer. In fact, it offers several explanations for the pain and suffering that exist in the world. I just don't think Ehrman found any of them to his liking. I can certainly understand his feelings.

We often have a young man in our home who is a self-declared atheist, or nontheist, as I like to say. He's a neighbor and a friend of the family. Not too long ago, my wife and daughters were playing cards with him at the kitchen table, and I was watching my grandson in the living room. We live in a small townhouse and everything is within hearing distance of everything else, so it's not like I was eavesdropping, at least, not intentionally.

But I did hear Cheryl, ever the smooth conversationalist, suddenly put our guest on the spot with this question: "So, I hear you don't believe in God anymore. Why is that?"

Politics and religion: the two topics you should never bring up when playing cards at the kitchen table. But this young man didn't seem to mind at all. I listened as he listed several reasons he no longer believes in God. Some of what he said I recognized as the arguments of the most famous nontheists of our time. That's because I've read their books, too. Hey, what can I say? I like to hear both sides of an issue.

Well, at some point in the conversation, the all-powerful/all-loving question was presented, and everyone at the table went silent. Then, Cheryl yelled to the living room, "Honey, can you please give this boy some answers?" In our house, I am chief dishwasher, garbage taker-outer, dog walker and, evidently, the primary theologian/philosopher on all questions that have stymied humankind throughout time.

"I can share with you some of the answers the Bible gives," I said to him, "but I can tell you right now that they are very unsatisfying." I am an honest theologian, if nothing else. Most of you who are still reading this chapter will probably agree with me as you work through the next few pages and subsequent chapter. You might even begin to understand the dissatisfaction and frustration that Dr. Ehrman felt as he read through the Bible for answers. You may even empathize with his heart's conclusions. On second thought, that's probably taking it a bit too far. After all, he's a distinguished professor at his university and an extremely successful author. He probably eats empathizers for lunch! Or so I've heard. Where do these vicious rumors get started, anyway?

~

One of the main explanations for pain and suffering in the world is that God is sovereign over all and, therefore, he controls (or at least allows) every detail of our lives. In other words, pain and suffering are here because God wants them here. The fancy definition of *sovereign* is that he has complete or supreme power over everything within his domain, which is everywhere, by the way. My definition of *sovereign* is that he can do whatever the heck he wants to do, whenever and wherever he chooses to do it. We humans just need to remember our place—that is, that he is God and we are not. Isaiah gives this analogy in his writings:

> Woe to those who quarrel with their Maker,
>> those who are nothing but potsherds among the
>> potsherds on the ground.
> Does the clay say to the potter,
>> "What are you making?" (Isaiah 45:9).

The answer is no, it does not.

Nowhere is this argument more clearly illustrated than in the book of Job. The story of Job is arguably one of the oldest in the Bible. Many scholars believe he was a contemporary or predecessor of Abraham. What's fascinating is that people were trying to answer the *why* questions even way back then, because that is what the entire book of Job is about.

If you're unfamiliar with the story, the opening scene is a conversation between God and Satan. God is bragging on Job:

> "Have you considered my servant Job? There is no one on earth like him; he is blameless and upright, a man who fears God and shuns evil" (Job 1:8).

Satan argues that it's because God has blessed Job. Then he dares God: "But now stretch out your hand and strike everything he has, and he will surely curse you to your face" (Job 1:11). God gives Satan his permission to do just that, evidently to prove him wrong. It's almost as if they make a wager. God is betting on Job; Satan is betting against him.

Let me pause here and vent for just a moment, if you don't mind. First, I would prefer that God never talk about me or mention my name to Satan. At first blush, it would seem to be a very positive thing that God was bragging on you. In the end, however, it apparently draws a whole lot of undue attention—the equivalent of drawing a target on someone's back. At least, that was certainly the outcome for Job. He experiences a perfectly orchestrated series of calamities designed by ... well, Satan himself—with God's permission, of course!

The second thing is, if this whole Parkinson's thing turns out to be a little bet between God and Satan, I'm probably going to be a little ticked off with God. Am I allowed to say that? Am I allowed to feel that way? I think that's only normal. That's what Job will eventually feel as well.

But back to Job chapter one: Job loses all of his livestock and his ten adult children in one day. The heartbreaking messages of each tragedy arrive one by one, each within a few minutes of the other. However, Satan is proven wrong. Job does not curse God to his face, but instead ends the chapter stoically declaring:

> "Naked I came from my mother's womb,
>   and naked I will depart.
> The Lord gave and the Lord has taken away;
>   may the name of the Lord be praised" (Job 1:21).

God is so proud that he brags on Job yet again in chapter 2:

> "Have you considered my servant Job? There is no one on earth like him; he is blameless and upright, a man who fears God and shuns evil. And he still maintains

his integrity, though you incited me against him to ruin him without any reason" (Job 2:3).

Those last three words are really troubling for me—"without any reason"—but that is part of the God-is-sovereign package deal. If God is sovereign, then not only does he control everything within his domain, but he also has no obligation whatsoever to explain his actions.

This time around God allows Satan to take away Job's health but not his life—and here's where the story starts to get personal for me—so Job is given some kind of disease. Again, this is with God's permission! In his case, Job is covered from head-to-toe with sores, and they so disfigure him that his friends can hardly recognize him. His wife tells him to go ahead and curse God and die. She was quite the encourager, right?

Chapter 3 opens with Job indeed cursing, not God, but the day he was born. In chapter 6, he prays for God to just end his life. In chapter 7, he asks God, "If I have sinned, what have I done to you?" and questions God with the verse with which we opened this chapter, "Why have you made me your target? Have I become a burden to you?" (Job 7:20).

You see, this was the line of reasoning proposed by Job's friends. The same friends who wisely sat silent for seven days at the beginning of their visit are now accusing Job of having sin in his life and saying that's the reason he is suffering. Of course, in the last chapter of the book, God tells those friends that they did not speak the truth, and he instructs them that if they want to be forgiven, they must ask Job to pray for them. They probably should have remained silent.

Meanwhile, Job's questions for God get progressively bolder. In chapter 10, he accuses God of knowing that he is innocent but making it impossible to be rescued from his hand. In chapter 13, he says he wants to speak to the Almighty directly and argue his case before him. Then, skipping ahead to chapter 31, he challenges God to weigh him in honest scales so he will know that Job is blameless. The insinuation is clearly that God is using some other kind of scales.

Then all heaven breaks loose. A storm rolls in—one translation says a whirlwind—and God speaks to Job out of the storm. It doesn't go well.

This is not a perfect analogy, but I can almost hear the voices of Tom Cruise and Jack Nicholson in the movie *A Few Good Men*, during the pivotal scene in which Colonel Jessup, played by Nicholson, shouts, "You want answers?" to which Lieutenant Kaffee, played by Cruise, responds, "I think I'm entitled to them." Then Jessup shouts louder, "You want answers?" and Kaffee shouts back, "I want the truth!" And Jessup responds with one of the most famous lines in all of filmdom: "You can't handle the truth!"

The analogy ends there, but I see Job as the one trying to get answers—because he believes he's entitled to them and, ultimately, the truth. God is the one who is finally roused to respond in chapter 38, where he quickly makes it clear that Job won't be able to handle the truth. Listen to God's opening line:

> "Who is this that obscures my plans with words
>   *without knowledge?*
> Brace yourself like a man;
>   I will question you,
>   and you shall answer me" (Job 38:2-3, italics mine).

OK, Job, you wanted to do this; let's do it!

Then, God begins to blast away:

"Where were you when I laid the earth's foundation?
    Tell me, if you understand.
Who marked off its dimensions? Surely you know"
(Job 38:4-5).

Who knew God could be so sarcastic? I think it's at this point that Job realizes he is out of his league, but he cannot stop the response that he has unleashed. For the next two chapters, God continues asking similar questions.

In chapter 40, God challenges Job again:

"Will the one who contends with the Almighty correct him?
    Let him who accuses God answer him!" (Job 40:2).

Job is done at this point and answers:

"I am unworthy—how can I reply to you?
    I put my hand over my mouth.
I spoke once, but I have no answer—
twice, but I will say no more" (Job 40:4-5).

But God is not done and fills another two chapters with questions that cannot be answered.

In some of the last words that Job utters in this story, he says to God:

"I know that you can do all things;
    no purpose of yours can be thwarted.
You asked, 'Who is this that obscures my plans without knowledge?'

Surely I spoke of things I did not understand,
things too wonderful for me to know" (Job
42:2-3).

In other words, I can't handle the truth!

In the end, God restores all of Job's fortunes and gives
him twice as much as he had before. He is given ten more
children, seven boys and three girls—and the girls are
considered to be the most beautiful women in the land. He
then lives to be 140 years old and sees four generations of
his descendants. There's no mention of his wife again.
Perhaps her punishment for telling him to curse God and
die in the beginning was to have to bear ten more children.

There are several details worth noting here. As far as
we know, God never tells Job the reasons why—or lack
thereof—he did what he did, and apparently Job does not
bring it up again. The loud-and-clear message that God
communicated to Job in the four chapters of unanswerable
questions was this: "When you know all that I know, then
you can question all that I do." I guess Job decided that he
was in over his head.

~

The God-is-sovereign explanation for pain and
suffering does account for the all-powerful attribute of
God. However, it does not seem to reflect in any way the
fact that God is all-loving. Instead, the God of Job comes
across as quite sarcastic and condescending. So, where's the
compassion? Where's the caring? Where's the love? The
message of the book of Job is that God is indeed
completely sovereign, but that's not all the Bible says about
God. He is much more than just the one attribute. We
need more than just the one perspective.

You see, the Bible is a collection of stories and encounters with God that people actually experienced. None of them are untrue nor meant to mislead, but none of them on their own can explain or describe God in all his fullness. In fact, neither can all of them put together. David says it very plainly in the Old Testament: "Great is the Lord and most worthy of praise; his greatness no one can fathom" (Psalm 145:3).

Paul echoes that thought in the New Testament:

"Oh, the depth of the riches of the wisdom and knowledge of God!
How unsearchable his judgments,
and his paths beyond tracing out" (Romans 11:33).

In other words, God is bigger than the theological statements we use to describe him. If we ever feel that we have described him perfectly with our words, we are no longer talking about God, but our own theological construct. He is, in a word, *unfathomable*!

Yet, having acknowledged the unfathomable quality of God, we must also say that the more perspectives we have on God, the more completely we may paint a portrait of him. In each story from the Bible, we see another aspect of who God is. In each encounter with him described within the biblical narratives, we walk away with a better understanding of what he's like. The portrait begins to take shape and we get a better understanding—but never fully, never completely. More is always better but never enough, if that makes sense.

So now, as we look to another possible explanation for the pain and suffering in this world, we go to another man's experience and perspective on God. As we do, we get another glimpse into the character and nature of God. The second story does not negate the first, but complements or supplements it. Now, turn from Job to Joseph.

~

    The second possible explanation for suffering is that God has a plan, and he is carrying out that plan in time and history. Because he is eternal and all-knowing, he can see the big picture that we can't see. Humans are limited by our linear perspective. We move through time chronologically—minute by minute, day by day, year by year. God, on the other hand, has no such limitations. He exists outside of time, and is, therefore, present simultaneously in the past, present, and future. It may hurt our brains to think about such things, but God seems fairly matter-of-fact when he describes himself in Isaiah: "I make known the end from the beginning, from ancient times, what is still to come" (Isaiah 46:10). In other words, he sees it all from start to finish—the big picture—as only he can do.

    Nowhere is the God-has-a-plan explanation seen more clearly than in Joseph's life story in the book of Genesis, chapter 37 to the end of the book. Joseph's life is filled with betrayal, abandonment, human trafficking, forced slavery, and, to top it all off, imprisonment for a crime he did not commit. It's all apparently for the sake of being in the right place at the right time later in his life, so that he could save his father and brothers from famine and starvation, not to mention the entire nation of Egypt.

    Surely, Joseph must have prayed many times for God to deliver him from his circumstances. However, God seemingly allowed him to endure suffering for decades for some greater good that Joseph would only understand later but have no way of knowing about while it was actually happening to him. The timing of Joseph's rise from prison to palace seemed to have more to do with the forgetfulness of a cupbearer who shared a cell with Joseph for a brief time than it did with God orchestrating event after event to a providential ending. Still, when it was all over, Joseph told his brothers: "You intended to harm me, but God intended it for good to accomplish what is now being done, the saving of many lives" (Genesis 50:20).

In his book, *Walking With God Through Pain and Suffering*, author and pastor Tim Keller talks about Joseph's unanswered prayers during the years he suffered without knowing why, and he offers this explanation: "Very often God does not give us what we ask for. Instead he gives us what we would have asked for if we had known everything he knows."

Only God, who knows the intricacies and the infinite details of not just of our lives but of all history, can see the end from the beginning and flawlessly manage the interconnectedness of it all. Sometimes, we may see the reasons for our suffering as we look back over our lives—hindsight is 20/20, they say—but sometimes we may not. I often think of it as a tapestry. On one side of the tapestry is a mess of threads and knots and colors with no apparent patterns or shapes. Flip it to the front side, however, and you see a beautiful work of art. Some of us don't get to see that beautiful flip side in our lifetime, sadly, but that does not make it untrue.

The idea of a tapestry came from listening to and reading the works of Corrie Ten Boom, in particular *The Hiding Place*, in which she tells how she and her family helped hide Jews during the Nazi Holocaust. Four of the Ten Boom family members gave their lives for the cause. Corrie herself survived three concentration camps and lived to tell the story. In her book, she includes this poem:

> My life is but a weaving between my God and me;
> I cannot choose the colors He worketh steadily.
> Oft' times He weaveth sorrow and I, in foolish pride,
> Forget He sees the upper, and I the under side.
> Not til the loom is silent and the shuttles cease to fly,
> Shall God unroll the canvas and explain the reason
> why.
> The dark threads are as needful in the Weaver's skillful
> hand,
> As the threads of gold and silver in the pattern He has
> planned.
> He knows, He loves, He cares, nothing this truth can
> dim
> He gives His very best to those who leave the choice to
> Him.

Joseph's story is a beautiful one when you get to the end where you can look back and see that the suffering was for a purpose that, at the time, only God could see. But when you don't know the ending and you're in the middle of whatever horrible circumstances you're going through, it all seems unfair and unjust.

If Joseph illustrates the God-has-a-plan explanation in the Old Testament, Hebrews 11 does so in the New Testament. It's the chapter often referred to as the "Hall of Faith." Many heroes of the Old Testament are described there. All the great names are included: Moses, Abraham, Isaac, Jacob, and Joseph, as well as others who "through faith conquered kingdoms, administered justice, and gained what was promised; who shut the mouths of lions, quenched the fury of the flames, and escaped the edge of the sword; whose weakness was turned to strength; and who became powerful in battle and routed foreign armies. Women received back their dead, raised to life again" (Hebrews 11:33-35).

All the people from this first list were blessed with miracles and supernatural interventions, obvious God-moments. We like to read about the first group. However, the writer continues with the stories of those who were not so blessed:

"There were others who were tortured, refusing to be released so that they might gain an even better resurrection. Some faced jeers and flogging, and even chains and imprisonment. They were put to death by stoning; they were sawed in two; they were killed by the sword. They went about in sheepskins and goatskins, destitute, persecuted and mistreated—the world was not worthy of them. They wandered in deserts and mountains, living in caves and in holes in the ground. These were all commended for their faith, yet none of them received what had been promised" (Hebrews 11:35-39).

Notice the words here. While the first group "gained what was promised," out of the second group, "none of them received what had been promised." The latter is not a verse we typically embroider and frame to put up in our kitchen, is it? I don't hear it preached or taught very often, either. We like to read through that one quickly.

But my question is: Why did some of them not receive what had been promised? The reason, according to the next verse, had nothing to do with the people who went through those difficult times. Instead, it apparently had something to do with the future: "None of them received what had been promised, since God had planned something better for us so that only together with us would they be made perfect" (Hebrews 11:39-40). The "us" in this passage would be the writer of Hebrews and his readers, New Testament believers. In other words, the people whose tragic stories are described in the second group of Hebrews 11 did not see a miracle or the answer for which they so desperately prayed apparently because of people who did not yet exist.

Again, we seem to be looking at the back side of a tapestry God is weaving and that is incomprehensible to us, for only he can see the interconnectedness of all the pieces, even thousands of years apart. Evidently, though, these men and women never lost hope, for the writer of Hebrews describes them as people whose faith should be commended and of whom the world was not worthy. They never, at least in this life, had the luxury of looking back and saying, "Ohhh, I see now!" as Joseph did. Maybe they got to see it later. The pastor of the church where I attend often says that the most spoken word in all of heaven will be, "Ohhh!" as we sometime see the reasons why. I'd sure like that to be true.

But until then, when we face inexplicable pain and suffering in our lives, and when we don't know the ending, there are some essential questions that theists must ask ourselves. Do we still trust God? Do we believe that he is good and loving? Do we believe that in every situation he is working for the good of those who love him and are called according to his purpose? (See Romans 8:28.) Unanswered prayers or tough times do not mean that God is not real, nor do they prove that he does not care or does not love us. Many people who come through difficult situations look back and see God's hand guiding them step-by-step and realize that they felt his presence to be more real than ever in their lives. The trying circumstances through which they traveled only highlighted the fact that God was with them. Their faith in God was affirmed, even strengthened.

That is one consolation that we often see in the Bible. God promises to be with us through whatever difficulties we must face. He shows us he loves us and cares for us by being there with us. Isaiah shares these words of comfort from God to his people in the Old Testament:

> But now, this is what the Lord says—
>> he who created you, Jacob,
>> he who formed you, Israel:
> "Do not fear, for I have redeemed you;
>> I have summoned you by name; you are mine.
> When you pass through the waters,
>> I will be with you;
> and when you pass through the rivers,
>> they will not sweep over you.
> When you walk through the fire,
>> you will not be burned;
>> the flames will not set you ablaze.
> For I am the Lord your God,
>> the Holy One of Israel, your Savior"
> (Isaiah 43:1-3).

If we return to the story of Joseph, we see a phrase repeated throughout chapter 39, in which he goes from slave to falsely accused criminal to prisoner: "the Lord was with him" (Genesis 39:2, 3, 21 and 23). Maybe that is what helped Joseph survive. Maybe that was the reason he didn't turn bitter and seek revenge on his brothers. Maybe that was what enabled him to say, "I suffered for a reason … for the saving of many lives."

If we accept the God-has-a-plan explanation for pain and suffering, then we believe that God sees the big picture of our lives and the lives of everyone else in the world throughout history, and that he is working out his plan for the maximum good of everyone concerned. We may see what he is doing during our lifetime as Joseph did in Genesis, or we may die before the promise comes, as did some of the heroes of the faith in Hebrews 11. But for all of us, God shows his love by being there with us. He has even been known to weep when we weep and be touched by our sadness, as we say elsewhere in this book. He becomes for us all our *Immanuel*—"God with us" (see Matthew 1:23).

So, does that mean that God allows us to go through hard times just to prove that he loves us and will be with us when we need him? I don't think so. I believe that he is weaving a wondrous work of art out of all our histories and that sometimes includes pain and suffering for one or a few for the salvation of many.

So, the God-has-a-plan explanation may account for both attributes of God, the fact that he is all-powerful—as in, he exercises control over every detail of our lives—and all-loving—the pain and suffering we experience in our lives is yet another chance for him to be with us.

There is one more major explanation that the Bible offers for the pain and suffering in this world. It may be the least satisfying of all yet the one closest to the truth. For that, we will devote another chapter.

Chapter Five
Why-ing Part 2

He will wipe every tear from their eyes. There will be no more death or mourning or crying or pain, for the old order of things has passed away. —Revelation 21:4

A campus pastor at one of the state universities in North Carolina recently contacted me. We're friends, and so he asked if I would come speak to a class of ministry interns, students who were planning to give one year of their lives to campus ministry after they graduate. I had taught some classes for him before, so I asked which class he wanted me to teach. He answered quickly, "Oh, it'll be a new one. I want you to teach on the problem of pain and why there is so much suffering in the world."

I asked, "And you thought of me?"

He said, "Well, yeah. I don't think anyone else could do it better." Evidently, I've become the poster boy for pain and suffering.

It was a six-hour class, and I actually enjoyed preparing for it. I had the interns divide and conquer several books prior to the class, including *The Problem of Pain* by C.S.

Lewis, *The Question That Never Goes Away* by Philip Yancey, *Walking With God Through Pain and Suffering* by Tim Keller, *If God is Good* by Randy Alcorn, and *God's Problem: How the Bible Fails to Answer Our Most Important Question—Why We Suffer* by Bart Ehrman. "Divide and conquer" meant that they all had to pick different books and give the class a report on what they'd read. I explained that they were to summarize their book for the students who didn't read it the way they wanted the other books summarized for them. I called it the "Golden Rule of Book Reports." What a teacher, right?

I listed all the Scriptures I could find on pain and suffering, and I broke them into categories: what I classified as the three major reasons that the Bible gives and all the minor ones, as well. I reread most of the books I had assigned to them and wrote out some great open-ended discussion questions to guide our conversation throughout the day. I was ready when the time finally came to teach the class. It was going to be a great day!

Within the first hour, I knew I was in trouble. My opening question was: What has been your closest brush or experience with the reality of pain and suffering? To my complete shock, none of these particular twenty-somethings had experienced anything truly painful in their lives—no tragic deaths of any of their relatives, no unexpected crises among their friends, no chronic diseases diagnosed within their families, no nasty divorces of their parents. Nothing! It was as if I got all the students who had lived inside a bubble for their first two decades.

As a result, this subject that fascinated me and consumed hours upon hours of my personal reflection time was all just a theoretical issue for them. "Well, you will experience some kind of pain and suffering at some point in your life," I said, sounding like some kind of doomsday prophet. All I was missing was a long beard and a sign that read, "The end is near!"

I continued: "When that day comes, what we're discussing today will really matter to you." And then, for the next five and a half hours, I talked. They listened politely, answered those great open-ended questions that I had prepared, and only nodded off occasionally when I went over the answers that the Bible gives for why we suffer.

When the class ended, one of them came up to me, thanked me for coming, and then said with heartfelt compassion, "You seem awfully worried about all this. I think you should lighten up a little bit and just enjoy life."

I think I said in return, "You know, you're right." But I was thinking, *You'll get this one day, kiddo.* Then I looked around for my "The end is near!" sign.

~

A third possible explanation for why there is pain and suffering in the world is this: God will one day take care of it all, but he's letting the consequences of our sinful nature and freedom of choice run their course until the end of history when he will make all things new again. The book of Revelation speaks of that exact scenario:

> Then I saw "a new heaven and a new earth," for the first heaven and the first earth had passed away, and there was no longer any sea. I saw the Holy City, the new Jerusalem, coming down out of heaven from God, prepared as a bride beautifully dressed for her husband. And I heard a loud voice from the throne saying, "Look! God's dwelling place is now among the people, and he will dwell with them. They will be his people,

and God himself will be with them and be their God. *'He will wipe every tear from their eyes. There will be no more death' or mourning or crying or pain,* for the old order of things has passed away." He who was seated on the throne said, "I am making everything new!" Then he said, "Write this down, for these words are trustworthy and true" (Revelation 21:1-5, italics mine).

Notice the first thing that God does in the new heaven and new earth: He wipes every tear from our eyes. I believe this wiping away of the tears affects our past, present, and future. The sad memories of the old order of things—of the first heaven and first earth, if you will—are erased with the promise of God attached: "I am making everything new!" The tears of that moment are brushed off our faces as well. And those of the future? It's not so much the tears themselves, but even the possibility of future tears is removed, for "there will be no more death or mourning or crying or pain." That's a pretty neat thought, come to think of it.

The next chapter reveals a little bit more:

Then the angel showed me the river of the water of life, as clear as crystal, flowing from the throne of God and of the Lamb down the middle of the great street of the city. On each side of the river stood *the tree of life,* bearing twelve crops of fruit, yielding its fruit every month. And the leaves of the tree are for the healing of the nations. *No longer will there be any curse.* The throne of God and of the Lamb will be in the city, and his servants will serve him. They will see his face, and his name will be on their foreheads. There will be no more night. They will not need the light of a lamp or the light of the sun, for the Lord God will give them light.

And they will reign for ever and ever. The angel said to me, "These words are trustworthy and true" (Revelation 22:1-6, italics mine).

The first time the tree of life was mentioned in the Bible was way back in Genesis chapters 2 and 3. In Genesis 2, it is one of the two named trees that were part of the garden of Eden: "In the middle of the garden were the tree of life and the tree of the knowledge of good and evil" (Genesis 2:9). If you know the story of Genesis, then you will recognize the second tree as the one Adam and Eve were commanded not to eat of its fruit. We'll circle back around to that little fiasco in a minute. What I want to emphasize is that we were always meant to eat from the first tree, both in Eden and in the new heaven and earth of Revelation. In the very beginning, though, we get kicked out of the garden because of this very tree and its potential. And I do mean kicked out, as in angels-with-flaming-swords kicked out. Why? Lest we (a.k.a. Adam and Eve) also "take from the tree of life and eat, and live forever" (Genesis 3:22). It seems we were always destined to live forever and would have, except for one little detail called "The Fall of Man." That little slip-up cost us Eden and so much more.

And there's another line we should note in Revelation 22. "No longer will there be any curse" (Revelation 22:3). What's the curse, you may ask? Well, in general, it's the set of consequences that came as a result of Adam and Eve's disobedience in the garden. God curses the serpent, then Eve, and finally Adam with very individualized punishments (Genesis 3:14-19) for each of their parts in the deed, but it affected the entire human race, too. Among other things, we, as the descendants of Adam and Eve, lost our right standing with God due to an inherited sinful nature. We were all condemned to experience physical death because of the same. (Gee, thanks, guys! There's so much more we could talk about here, but I'm trying to stay focused.) In this new heaven and earth, however, the writer of Revelation tells us the curse will be lifted and those two entire-human-race consequences are gone. We are once again in right standing with God—hey, he's actually going to be our neighbor (see Revelation 21:3)—and we will no longer experience death, but instead will live forever. That's the way it was before the fall in Eden and the way it will be again in the new heaven and new earth. In fact, in my Bible, the passage from Revelation 22 is subtitled: "Eden restored." In other words, we're going back to what God had originally planned for us all along, it would seem.

All of that is my attempt to say this: We are now living between the two Edens, if you will. We are living between the two appearances of the tree of life. We are living between the perfect place that God made for humankind in the beginning and the new version of that perfect place planned for some point in our future, where—once again—there will be no more pain or suffering, evil or sin, death or dying, or mourning or crying. That sounds awfully good, does it not?

But we're not there yet, we might not be there for a while, and in between those two perfect places is a whole lot of imperfection. That is to say, all those things that will not be in the new heaven and earth are still here now in abundance. Why? I believe that God is allowing us to go with the consequences of our freewill choices. When I say *our*, I mean those of the entire human race and of everyone who has lived on the planet throughout history. One person may be making all the right choices he or she can possibly make, but when his or her path crosses the path of someone who is doing the opposite, pain and suffering may be involved.

What about miracles, divine intervention, answered prayer? Are those still a possibility? Yes! But by their very nature, true miracles are few and far between, except when we're talking about the life of Jesus. His ministry on earth seemed to be full of them, but could we chalk that up to special circumstances, such as being the Son of God? In the rest of the Bible, there appears to be wider gaps between miracles. They may seem to take place on every page of the Bible, but often there are days, weeks, months, years, decades, and sometimes centuries represented by the simple turn of a page. I am by no means counting out miracles. I'm just not sure we should look for them every day. God could do that, of course, but does he?

What about natural disasters that are not the result of freedom of choice? Like hurricanes, earthquakes, and tsunamis? Well, there's another part of the curse mentioned in the Bible. It's a curse upon the earth itself, sometimes referred to as *creation*. It's alluded to in Genesis 3 and Paul writes about it at length in Romans 8:

> For the creation waits in eager expectation for the children of God to be revealed. For the creation was subjected to frustration, not by its own choice, but by the will of the one who subjected it, in hope that the creation itself will be liberated from its bondage to decay and brought into the freedom and glory of the children of God. We know that the whole creation has been groaning as in the pains of childbirth right up to the present time. Not only so, but we ourselves, who have the firstfruits of the Spirit, groan inwardly as we wait eagerly for our adoption to sonship, the redemption of our bodies (Romans 8:19-23).

The creation was subjected to frustration by God, Paul says, and put in bondage to decay. We see this in the universe winding down, our sun getting older, and the earth beneath us slowly deteriorating. And all the while the earth is longing for the same redemption for which we humans await. The new heaven and new earth? I think so. Old Mother Earth, it seems, is looking for a better place, too.

The God-will-one-day-take-care-of-it-all explanation is a cop-out, my nontheist friends would say. They would explain that I am simply denying the reality of something they know to be true: the nonexistence of God. God, however, gave humans free will and has never forced anyone to believe in him or follow his ways. He has done this since the very beginning of human history, so why would he change course now? He is all-powerful and will prove that one day, for all the world to see. He is also all-loving and has already proven that. As the Apostle John writes in 1 John: "This is how God showed his love among us: He sent his one and only Son into the world that we might live through him. This is love: not that we loved God, but that he loved us and sent his Son as an atoning sacrifice for our sins" (1 John 4:9-10). That one act of the God-became-human Jesus stands out in history as the indisputable moment that God proved that he loved us ... and loves us, still.

~

So, in my humble opinion, those are the Bible's big three answers to the *why* question. See what I mean by *unsatisfying*? None of them is a perfect answer, filling in all the doubts and arguments and protests we may have in our heads or hearts. Perhaps it's a combination of all three combined.

If we applied all of the above to my Parkinson's diagnosis, then the answer to the *why* question would sound something like this: I have Parkinson's because I live in a world full of sickness and disease and I was one of the unlucky ones that happened to get this particular ailment. I'm looking forward to the day when God gets rid of all this stuff in the future, but until that day comes, I'm going to shuffle on. Could he have prevented it? Could he heal me from it now? Yes and yes. I'm still hoping for a miracle, but I know he sees the big picture in time and history that I cannot see. Who knows? Maybe my battle with Parkinson's is meant to inspire someone else or prepare my friends for the curve ball that life will soon throw them or maybe it's nothing so obvious at all, but one day I'll know and say, "Ohhh ... now I get it." But in the meantime, I'm discovering that I'm praying more and feeling God's loving presence nearer to me than I ever have before. I'm realizing that his grace really is sufficient for me. Sometimes, I can sense him shuffling right along beside me. Ultimately, I know that he is in control of every detail of my life. Nothing takes him by surprise nor catches him off guard. Maybe he allowed this chronic disease into my life because he wanted me to know what I would do if he did not respond in the affirmative to my prayers. As a matter of fact, I would like to know that answer, too. I'm living it out every day.

Now, is that such a terrible way to process what is happening to me? I don't think so. It's allowing for the God-will-one-day-take-care-of-it-all, God-has-a-plan, and God-is-sovereign explanations to complement and supplement one another as pieces of the puzzle that is my life. God can see the final picture that he's working toward because he's got the puzzle box. I'm just trying to match pieces of similar color, pattern, or shape. I look around me and see all the pieces yet to be placed, and I think it's going to take a lifetime to finish this. God is probably thinking, "Well, look who just caught up!" He can be sarcastic sometimes, you know.

~

I'm not claiming that the three explanations I have are the only ones the Bible offers. There are several other possibilities that could also be considered, such as:

God wants to use me for the spiritual benefit of others (Philippians 1:19-30).
God is teaching me or showing me how to comfort others (2 Corinthians 1:3-7).
God is trying to produce in me perseverance, character, and hope (Romans 5:1-5).
God is trying to teach me humility (2 Corinthians 12:1-7).
God is trying to teach me obedience (Hebrews 5:7-10).
God is making me more like Jesus (Philippians 3:10-14, Romans 8:16-18, 1 Peter 2:21).
God is disciplining me because he loves me (Hebrews 12:5-11).
God is seeking to bring glory to his name (1 Peter 1:6-7, Matthew 5:16, John 9:1-5).

While these reasons may all seem to be totally unrelated and random, I do notice a common thread weaving itself through all but the final two verses. Do you see it? In each of the other passages, God is attempting to transform the character of the people he is allowing to experience pain and suffering—to produce in them, among other things, concern and compassion for others, perseverance, humility, obedience, and so on—in a word, to make them more like Christ. That would tie in with an idea and a verse we have already observed a few chapters back in this book: "For those God foreknew he also predestined to be conformed to the image of his Son, that he might be the firstborn among many brothers and sisters" (Romans 8:29). That's the end goal God has in mind for everyone who follows him: to conform him or her to the image of Christ. But why?

In 2013, Pope Francis, in one of his morning homilies, made an interesting comment that might just answer the question. He said, "The whole journey of life is a journey of preparation for heaven. [Jesus is] preparing our ability to enjoy the chance, our chance to see, to feel, to understand the beauty of what lies ahead, of that homeland toward which we walk." I like that idea. Heaven will certainly be a much more enjoyable place if everyone who goes there walks, talks, and lives with the same grace, mercy and compassion that Jesus demonstrated while he was on earth. Wouldn't you agree?

So, could another possible reason why we suffer in this life be because God is preparing us for heaven? In other words, could God be transforming us into the kind of people that would make heaven *heaven*?

I once heard someone tell the story of a man who asked God to give him a glimpse of heaven and hell. God showed him two doors. He opened the first one, and the smell of a delicious stew filled the air. Everyone inside, however, was thin and unhealthy and looked to be starving. They all held spoons with very long handles, longer than their arms, which made it impossible to dip into the stew and back to their mouths. God then closed the door and said, "That was hell."

Then, he opened the next door, and again the smell of a delicious stew filled the air. These people had the very same long-handled spoons, but in this place everyone was healthy and happy and appeared to be well-nourished. "This is heaven," God said.

The man asked what the difference was, and God explained, "The difference is love. Love has taught those in heaven to be concerned for others, so these people have learned to dip into the stew and feed each other."

That's a fictional story, of course, but it makes the point. Maybe we should add one more official possibility to the reasons *why*: God is preparing us for heaven. Sometimes, on this side of heaven, it feels like we are going through hell to get there, but will it not be worth it? Paul says something like that in his letter to the Romans: "I consider that our present sufferings are not worth comparing with the glory that will be revealed in us" (Romans 8:18). I really want to believe that with all my heart.

~

I want to end this chapter with a vision I had. Maybe a better word would be daydream. I'm not claiming it was some kind of special revelation from God during which I heard audible voices and saw images flashing across my bedroom ceiling. That would be weird and more than a little bit spooky. I'm not saying people can't have those, but God probably knows I would be really freaked out. I prefer something slightly less theatrical.

Sadly, this whatever-you-want-to call-it came to me with the death of a young man who finally lost his battle with acute lymphocytic leukemia. Dwight, or DJ, was a handsome young man with an enthusiasm for life that was absolutely contagious, a big smile that would warm your soul, and an incredibly strong faith in God, despite all that he went through. And he endured quite a bit, including a bone marrow transplant with stem cells from an umbilical cord and the removal, reengineering and reinfusion of his T cells to fight off the leukemic cells. He participated in clinical trials at Children's Hospital of Philadelphia, Duke University School of Medicine, the National Institutes of Health, and Cleveland Clinic. He went back and forth between remission and relapse for several years before he succumbed to the disease at age 22.

I met him when he was a teenager, and I have vivid memories of him standing up in our church and inspiring everyone with his rap songs that praised God for the times he was in remission:

Remember me laying in the hospital,
Remember me refusing to eat food,
Remember me begging for the chemo,
And now I'm standing here thanking my hero.

On the morning of his funeral, I couldn't shake the picture in my head of DJ's big smiling face. The picture became a scene, and I watched as the movie began to play out in my mind.

Dwight was walking up to the entrance to heaven alone. None of the usual props were there. There were no pearly gates or a big desk with a book of approved names. Saint Peter wasn't guarding the door. There was just one, solitary figure waiting for Dwight: It was Jesus.

For as far as you could see, there were rolling hills of whiteness, everywhere. The ground on which they walked was covered with white, too, and it wasn't snow or clouds. I couldn't tell what it was. As Dwight grew closer, Jesus started running toward him and wrapped his arms around him in a giant bear hug. They both began to weep.

They held that embrace for a good long while, and, when they finally pulled back, Jesus looked into his eyes and said, "I've been waiting a long time for this day. I am so glad you are finally here." They both began to weep again, until Jesus pulled back once more and with his thumbs gently wiped the tears from Dwight's eyes.

A peace came over Dwight's face, and they both smiled. Jesus, patting him on the shoulder, asked, "Are you ready for a personal tour of heaven?"

Dwight laughed: "I can't wait!"

"Before the tour," Jesus explained, "there is a receiving line we have to do with everyone whose life you touched or will touch. You'll enjoy that. Then, I'll give you the tour."

Suddenly, Dwight looked down and saw that Jesus was wearing a bright orange "Fight with Dwight" t-shirt, something many of us had worn during the days Dwight was still with us. When Jesus saw that he had noticed, he said, "You fought the good fight, Dwight. Well done!"

As they both turned to walk away, Jesus stopped Dwight and asked, "Wait. Do you have your list of questions? All the things you wanted to ask me when you got here?"

Dwight reached into his pocket and pulled out the list, written on white paper. At that same moment, Dwight's foot moved and he heard the sound of paper crinkling underneath his shoe. He sees what all the whiteness really is. Under their feet, and extending for acres in every direction, forming hills and valleys and the very road that they are standing on, are all of the *why* lists for everyone who had ever come through the entryway from the beginning of time. Dwight realized that he didn't care about his list anymore, either. He grinned at Jesus, wadded up the list, and threw it as far as he could throw into the piles and piles of crumpled up papers.

"I'm ready for that receiving line," Dwight said, beaming that contagious smile of his.

As they walked out of sight, Jesus' hand was resting on Dwight's shoulder. "I should warn you. Yours is rather lengthy," he said, "but that's a good thing."

~

I don't spend my every waking moment thinking about the *why* question. I'm convinced that it's above my pay grade. I'm also convinced of a few other things. That whole "wiping away of tears" will be significant for us. I'm just speculating, but I believe it will somehow heal our memories so the sadness, suffering, or whatever we came through won't be able to hurt us anymore. I'm convinced that once we're in the presence of Jesus, most of us, if not all of us, will throw away the list of questions. It seems to matter now because we're in the middle of our seemingly unfair or unjust circumstances, but I believe the reality of Jesus standing there ready to receive us will be so overwhelming that we won't be able to think about anything else.

One last thing: I know the Bible says there will be no more crying in heaven and that in my little scene above, both Jesus and Dwight wept. Well, technically, they were at the entryway into heaven. Heaven itself was just on the other side of all that paper. Second, I think Jesus can break the rules anytime he chooses. It's his house, his rules, and all that.

Chapter Six
Writing

I, Paul, write this greeting in my own hand, which is the
distinguishing mark in all my letters. This is how I write.
—2 Thessalonians 3:17

Evidently, Paul did not write all of his epistles. Oh, the
words are his, inspired by God, we believe. But with some
of the letters, for reasons not entirely known to us, he chose
to dictate to a scribe. He did that for his epistle to the
Romans, for example, and Tertius, the scribe who helped
him, adds his own little note of greeting to the letter (see
Romans 16:22). He probably felt he deserved a little credit
after transcribing sixteen chapters.

We don't know the name of the scribe who helped
with the second letter to the Thessalonians, but we do
know that one verse short of being done, Paul apparently
took the pen and wrote this little note: "I, Paul, write this
greeting in my own hand, which is the distinguishing mark
in all my letters. This is how I write" (2 Thessalonians
3:17). I love this personal touch. Paul must have had a very
distinctive script, and, either apologetically or

unapologetically, he points to it and says, "This is how I write."

He inserts another handwritten greeting at the end of Colossians and yet another at the end of his letter to the Galatians. In the latter, he makes it known: "See what large letters I use as I write to you with my own hand!" It would appear that Paul did not suffer from Parkinson's. For many of us with Parkinson's, there is a symptom called *micrographia*, which is extremely small handwriting, to the point that it's almost unreadable. As a teacher, I've seen it affect my lettering more and more. On the whiteboard in my classroom, I start out writing large letters and end up making excuses. "Sorry, guys, but some days this is how I write."

~

In preparation for my deep brain stimulation surgery, I was required to have a neuropsychological evaluation. A friend who had already been through the DBS process said the doctors wanted to test my IQ before and after the installation of the stimulator to see if there was any leakage of intelligence during the surgery itself. He winked and said, "They want to make sure you have a high enough IQ that you could afford to drop a couple of points and still function." This is the same friend who had a full head of hair grow back after his surgery, while my bald spots just became more obvious. If he weren't such a nice guy, I'd really dislike him.

I went in for the neuropsych evaluation, and it wasn't what I expected. For two and a half hours, I drew designs on paper with colored pencils, put puzzles together, figured out patterns on cards, and tried to remember lists of names, numbers, and letters. On some of the tests, I seemed to do well. Some left me searching for words. When I struggled, I admitted it right away, and the psychometrist would tell me I was doing better than I probably thought I was doing.

What felt like brain games actually were tests carefully designed to measure my thinking skills and abilities. Many of those tests had fancy-sounding names complete with their own acronyms, such as auditory consonant trigrams (ACT), digit vigilance test (DVT), and controlled oral word association test (COWAT-FAS). Some of them had not-so-fancy names, such as the cookie theft story, the Boston naming test and the clock drawing. I'm sure the latter were just as important as the former in the grand scheme of things. After going through dozens of these tests, I went home frustrated that I couldn't think of more words that started with the letter A. For some reason, I froze on that question. I could have used a good episode of *Sesame Street* right about then!

I came back the next week for my test results. At first, I was flattered. I got superior ratings in several areas, including vocabulary, verbal abstract reasoning, and nonverbal abstract reasoning. The doctor bragged on me for a few minutes, and then she let me down easy. I was comparatively weak in several areas, too: word generation, working memory, and processing speed. I say *comparatively*. These areas had average scores, but they should have been much higher based on my other scores.

She summarized for us: I was an educated, intelligent man with an extensive vocabulary and excellent reading and writing skills, all of which helped me to mask partially the fact that I could not always access the knowledge in my brain as quickly as I would like or as I had perhaps been able to do before. She was exactly right, of course. I knew that I now sometimes stumbled with my words, trying to think of a synonym for a word I cannot, for the life of me, recall.

Cheryl looked at the doctor intently, and then, carefully choosing her words, said: "So, are you going to tell us anything new?" She looked at me and winked. I thought about making a smart remark back to her, but at that particular moment I couldn't think of anything with just the right amount of sting. As usual, it would come to me later.

This was, indeed, old news. I knew quite well that when my meds were active and giving me the maximum symptoms relief possible, I did much better in the problem areas the doctor had mentioned—and significantly worse when they wore off.

~

I have noticed a significant difference between writing this book and writing my first one. I wrote the first draft of *Shuffle* in two months. I remember the start date was October 25, and I finished the last chapter on Christmas day that same year. I still had the editing, rewriting, and publishing steps to go through, so it would not be released for three more months, on March 25, to be exact. But the writing went fairly smoothly, with no problem with word generation, processing speed, and so forth. I had a goal of 500 words a day, and most days I wrote much more.

But that was a year and a half ago. There's a noticeable difference now, despite the fact that with both books the chapter ideas came to me all at once, along with the alliterated chapter titles—last time with the letter H and this time with the letter W. So, what's the difference? Plain and simple, I'm not reaching 500 words a day, anymore.

Earlier on with my Parkinson's, I had the luxury of generating that many words without a problem, with what the neuropsychologist would have called *fluency*. I like to call it *fluidity*, as in when the words seem to flow out like a river, gushing forward with all the right ideas, perfect phrases, and corresponding story lines. Now, however, I feel like the reservoir is still full but not all the floodgates are open. In practical terms, it's making me think and write a little slower. I can still do occasional 500-word days and sometimes even more if I feel inspired but, quite frankly, inspiration usually means insomnia and may cost me half the night. I have to choose between fluidity at 2 a.m. or lucidity the next day. I do not always choose wisely.

Lack of fluidity also means that when I speak publicly, I rely on manuscripts. I recently spoke at the high school graduation for the academy where I work. I wrote the speech out entirely, memorized most of it, but dared not rely on my memory alone. I had every word in front of me, just in case. I did the same for a wedding I just officiated, word for word, just in case. It's my way of working around the effects of my Parkinson's and not letting it take away a few of the things I enjoy doing. I've had that philosophy since the beginning of this experience.

~

My processing speed has also affected one of the habits I talked about in *Shuffle*. I said that I was an avid reader, trying to read one book a week or a total of fifty-two for the year. I was convinced—and I still am—that reading is one of the ways I can keep my mind sharp. Plus, as I tell my students all the time, we all need to be lifelong learners and reading is one of the ways we can do that. However, my ability to read through a book quickly seems to be slightly diminished. The last year I hit fifty-two was the year before my first book was published, and, if I remember correctly, I only made it that year because I was ahead of the count before I started writing *Shuffle*. The next year, I only got twenty books read, and this year will probably end with about fifteen. The first year I kept my book diary I had only twelve. That was eighteen years ago, but I may be back to that number soon.

But I refuse to quit or say I'm done. If twelve is my new number, back by popular demand, then twelve it shall be, with occasional bursts up to eighteen or so. I will never stop reading, and I'm allowing myself the privilege of listening to audio books during my commute or when I travel. I'm counting those as well. My latest? Carmine Gallo's *Talk Like TED: The 9 Public-Speaking Secrets of the World's Top Minds*. That's what I'm striving for, after all, to stay among the world's top minds, although I'm toward the back of the pack, surely.

There's another thing I'm doing to stay sharp mentally: I'm writing. While I've already confessed that the words come to me more slowly, I consider the whole process of putting my thoughts into written words to be curiously therapeutic and one of the things that has kept me sane for the last few years. As a friend told me a few years back: "You've read enough books to know what good books are supposed to sound like. Now, write your own." That message arrived by text on Friday, October 25. Do your recognize the date? Well, about five months later, *Shuffle* was born.

In the acknowledgements, I thanked my good friend with these words: "You started all this with a simple text, and I am forever grateful. You lit a fire in me that I cannot seem to put out." Nowadays, I'm writing every chance I get, whether it's a book, magazine article, devotional guide, sermon manuscript, or graduation speech. I haven't started a blog, yet, but that's probably in my future. I even have an idea for a sci-fi novel, but when I explained the plot to my editor, she asked if I'd eaten too much pizza the night before.

During the rewrites of the first book, I was bugging my editor every day to see where she was in the process. Finally, she said: "I'll tell you when I'm done. You'll be the first to know, I promise. Why don't you go out and start another book, a nice, long one with lots of pages?" Looking back, I think she was being sarcastic, but I took her words to heart. The next day I started writing a 365-page devotional guide for my high school students. It's nowhere close to publication, but I enjoy working on it every chance I get.

Then, there's this book. It had a friend-inspired beginning, too. A few months before my DBS surgery, one of my seminary professors called to see how I was doing health-wise. I described the upcoming DBS process and told him that I appreciated his concerns and prayers. He also shared some good news concerning *Shuffle*: Many of my stories in that first book were based on our years as missionaries in Costa Rica and Honduras and I talked about everything from culture shock to language learning, so the book now was required reading for all missionaries our sending agency commissioned to serve in Central and South America. I was honored, to put it mildly, and agreed to participate in an online forum with missionary candidates.

He asked if I was close to finishing my Master's program through the seminary. I laughed. I'd been working on my degree since my early days as a missionary, when the school offered one graduate course each summer for those of us overseas. Then, during my every-fifth-year furloughs back in the States, I would take as many courses as time and money would allow, slowly inching toward completion.

I explained that I had completed my coursework and only lacked the final field education research project, a paper reflecting my integration of the knowledge I had learned as a seminary student within my current ministry context. The FERP is usually about the length of a thesis but designed specifically for religious personnel already working in places of leadership and ministry. I told him I hadn't really started on the FERP and, because of time and money, didn't know when I could do so.

"Unless," I said, "the seminary would count as an equivalency a book that is now required reading for all missionary candidates commissioned to Central and South America."

We both laughed, and he answered, "I'm glad you're in good spirits. We'll be praying for the DBS to be a complete success."

Two days later, he called me with great news: "I talked with the Academic Dean, and we've decided to let your 130-page book count as your FERP. The only catch is that you would have to, number one, identify 1,500-plus pages you read in preparation for writing *Shuffle*. Number two, you would have to write a fifteen- to twenty-page paper that gives the background that led to writing the book, the key biblical and theological truths it espouses, and its impact on your life and ministry." He went on to say that they had secured a scholarship to pay the tuition.

I couldn't believe what I was hearing. I was speechless—and not just because of my poor word-generation skills nowadays. I expressed my deepest gratitude and said that I would start on the reading list and the reflection paper right away.

The first part was easy, because I keep a diary of every book I read. The pages I'd read in preparation for the book came in just under 3,000 total, so that was easy enough.

And, then, when I started writing the reflection paper, I had twenty-five pages before I even turned around, and that was just two weeks in. I contacted the professor and asked him for the absolute maximum page count for the project, because evidently I loved the sound of my own typing.

He said that I could go as long as I needed, but I had to make it good. I turned in my thirty-eight-page reflection paper two weeks later. I hadn't meant to double the numbers for both assignments, but that's part of the point I'm making.

This newfound passion is both cathartic and a source of great joy. I sometimes lose track of time as I write and suddenly realize that I've been at it for hours. I'm reminded of the line from the film *Chariots of Fire,* in which Eric Liddell is explaining to his sister, Jenny, why he feels like he must first run in the Olympics before going to China as a missionary: "I believe that God made me for a purpose … for China. But he also made me fast. And when I run I feel his pleasure. To give it up would be to hold him in contempt."

I feel like that sometimes, not about running, but about writing. When I write, I feel his pleasure. I don't throw my head back and look toward heaven as I type, like Eric did when he ran, nor do I hear the cool theme music in the background. Maybe I'll start playing it, though.

The end of the story is that the book and the paper completed the requirements for my Master's degree and sparked the idea for this sequel. Almost as soon as I handed in the paper for the research project, I started writing these pages. I was invited to fly to the seminary and walk across the stage to receive my degree, but I was right in the middle of the DBS process and I thought it would look a little strange to go up with two freshly drilled holes in my head. I was just as thrilled to receive it by mail. Besides, it got me back to my writing more quickly.

~

I recently read an article in the *New York Times* entitled, "Writing Your Way to Happiness." The author of the piece was Tara Parker-Pope, a regular contributor to the paper's column, "Well." The gist of the article was that expressive writing had proven to be beneficial to patients in many ways: as a mood improver, stress reducer, memory booster, and so forth. As I researched this idea more, I found all kinds of scientific research that supports writing as a valid therapy.

I'm convinced that just the process of writing down our thoughts can help us not only cope with our less-than-ideal circumstances but also enable us to see where we might need to adjust our thinking and behavior. It sometimes may even move us toward a greater sense of happiness. For example, Parker-Pope referred to a study of 120 married couples. Some were asked to write about a marital conflict that they had experienced but to do so from an outsider's point of view. The rest of the couples did not do the write-up. Do you want to guess which group showed measurable improvement in their relationships? The first group did, of course. Writing about the conflict enabled them to see their words and actions from the vantage point of a neutral observer. It allowed them to see their individual mistakes and to adjust accordingly.

How could just writing do that for us? I believe that as our thoughts flow down through our hands and fingers, whether we write them out or type them onto a screen, our mind has to do some organizational work with those thoughts—classifying them, collecting them, sorting them—so that we can articulate clearly and succinctly what's in our mind. The process of writing itself forces us to think about what we think, if you will.

Elizabeth Sullivan is a licensed marriage and family therapist from San Francisco. Margarita Tartakovsky interviewed her for the article "The Power of Writing" on PsychCentral.com. Sullivan put it this way: "Most of us do not think in complete sentences but in self-interrupted, looping, impressionistic cacophony. Writing helps us track our spinning thoughts and feelings, which can lead to key insights. ... We come to know who we really are in the present moment." The process can be enlightening for us, in other words, and for others if we go public.

I'm not suggesting that everyone has to publish a book, post a blog, or print a magazine article, although those are worthy objectives and they create awareness of what it's like to live with Parkinson's or anything else we are experiencing. But something as simple as journaling can be just as therapeutic for the one who is writing. Even if no one else ever sees our words—if we never publish, post, or print—we have benefited from the task of organizing our thoughts and maybe catching a glimpse of what we really think and feel for the first time.

When I wrote *Shuffle*, I described a conversation I had with a friend who said that her husband had basically given up trying to beat Parkinson's and had succumbed to the depression he had been battling for years. He had stopped doing any sort of exercise or physical therapy, was bedridden, unable to speak, and he rarely left his home. She had concluded: "I just don't think he cared for or loved me enough to keep on trying. I guess I wasn't worth the effort."

That conversation had prompted me to write my Parkinson's Partner Pledge to Cheryl, which, by the way, was a total surprise to her. It's the only part of *Shuffle* she didn't proof beforehand, so she didn't actually read the pledge until she was looking through the first printed copy of the book. She cried. If you know Cheryl, crying's not too unusual, but I was thrilled that we kept that a secret until the book's release.

But back to the couple I was describing above. There's no doubt in my mind that the husband was probably suffering from depression. At least half of all patients with Parkinson's disease do. There's also no doubt that he was in the advanced stage of Parkinson's. In comparison, I'm still in the mild stage. (For more information on the stages, you can visit the Parkinson's Disease Foundation website at pdf.org/en/progression_parkinsons.) Not everyone will progress to the advanced stage, but he certainly did. The symptoms would have included great difficulty walking, confinement to either a wheelchair or bed most of the day, not able to live alone, assistance needed with all daily activities, and significant cognitive problems. There are effective therapies to ease symptoms and make it possible for people with Parkinson's to live well at every stage, but his depression may have dissuaded him from exploring those options.

He died the same month and year that I finished *Shuffle*, but he did have some good days in those final years. I know at least on some of those days, he spent part of his time writing. Well, actually, he typed—slowly—but he did it. In a little journal called *A Father's Legacy: A Lasting Heritage for Your Children*, he wrote this first entry: "I can't write very good so I will put my entry on the computer and leave it here." He actually ended up printing out his words and placing them in the appropriate journal pages. He had an entry for almost every page in the first half of the journal.

When the journal question asked when he met his

wife, he typed these words: "I was working at the little country store when I was about sixteen. It must have been 1954 or 55. This man came into the store. He looked like a gangster, the type with a cigarette hanging from his lips and a felt hat with the brim turned down in the front. He went to the pop box and got out a Pepsi and came over to the counter where I was. He said to me give me a pack of Luckies (Lucky Strike Cigarettes) and I will take this Pepsi for my little girl as he motioned toward the door. I looked over at the door. There stood the prettiest girl I had ever seen. She had long hair and a beautiful smile. It was Jo."

He later talks about how he and his friend took Jo and her sister horseback riding and the mom came out on the porch when they were done and invited the boys to church. He ran home to change clothes, came back, and went to church with her family. He himself had not been in church for about three years, but in his words: "I really didn't care. I was with the girl I loved. After that we dated for a while, and then we didn't, then we got back together. And the rest is history … we got married in that little church, in 1958."

He finished about half the journal before he couldn't type any more, but he seemed to answer all the questions that had anything to do with his wife: getting engaged, buying the ring, renting their first apartment, expecting their first baby. But it's the last entry that tugged at my heart. The question at the top of the page was: "What do I love best about your Mom now?"

These were the final words that he typed out: "I am answering this after we have been married almost forty-four years. I still think your Mother is more beautiful now than she was then. My heart goes flippity flop when I kiss her. I know I love her more than then. I am sorry for my illness. It is very hard to show affection when you are in pain all the time. I don't know if anyone knows how much I suffer."

My heart is saddened when I think about how much pain he was obviously enduring there in the end, but even more so to realize how much this man loved his wife—but she didn't know it and he couldn't show it like he wanted to. But he wrote it all down and his words reach out even now to touch and mend and heal and confirm what was always there.

Thanks to Ray, I have a new line to use for Cheryl: "My heart goes flippity flop when I kiss you." She's probably going to cry again.

~

Writing *Shuffle* helped me do what I'm talking about here. Thinking through the things I wanted to say in that book was my first attempt at collecting my thoughts. There were scribbled notes on napkins, empty envelopes, and random scraps of paper scattered across the surface of my desk. The notes that were thematically connected I sorted into eight separate piles and then gave names—a.k.a. chapter titles—to those piles. Once I had the chapter titles, I began to think of Bible verses and personal stories that would appropriately reflect and properly illustrate the main ideas the piles represented. Then I started writing with every chapter already basically outlined. All that was left to do was find the best possible words to express all those ideas.

Wait, am I describing what actually happened with *Shuffle* or the organizational process that we all go through when we write? The answer is yes. So, start a journal, write a book, or create a blog. And here's to your health and happiness.

Chapter Seven
Working

The Lord God took the man and put him in the Garden of Eden
to work it and take care of it.
—Genesis 2:15

Genesis 1 and 2 tell the story of the creation of the heavens and the earth, and all things living, including humans. They also describe Eden before the Fall—that is, before Adam and Eve sinned against God and got kicked out of the Garden. That means that everything described in those two chapters were the way things were supposed to be in God's original plan for humankind. We were supposed to eat of the Tree of Life and live forever. Apparently, we were meant to walk around naked and unashamed. And from chapter 3 we also learn that evidently God regularly walked through the Garden in the cool of the day as if they were all good, good friends.

The verse for this chapter is part of that before-they-got-kicked-out-of-the-Garden narrative as well. It says: "The Lord God took the man and put him in the Garden of Eden to work it and take care of it" (Genesis 2:15). That means that God intended for humanity (Adam) to work from the very beginning of time. Working for survival and/or for a living was always part of the plan for human beings. Some people say that the idea of work came from the curse that God pronounced upon Adam after he sinned in Genesis 3. But here in Genesis 2, Adam had a job already, to work the Garden and take care of it. No, what changed after he sinned was the intensity of that work.

> Cursed is the ground because of you;
> through painful toil you will eat food from it
> all the days of your life.
> It will produce thorns and thistles for you,
> and you will eat the plants of the field.
> By the sweat of your brow
> you will eat your food
> until you return to the ground,
> since from it you were taken;
> for dust you are
> and to dust you will return (Genesis 3:17-19).

Those phrases such as "painful toil" and "sweat of your brow" are the dead giveaways. Adam was always supposed to work. But when he got kicked out of Eden, now he was going to have do some sweating.

~

I've had to have a job since shortly after I turned sixteen years old. That's because my mom and dad "gave" me a brand-new car at the beginning of my junior year of high school. It was October 20, 1978. I remember the day well. I had just washed the family station wagon to use for my date that night, when my dad drove up in a bright-red

Honda Civic, pulled up behind the station wagon, stepped out of the car and handed me the keys.

"Thought you might like to take this car instead," he said. "It's yours."

I yelled, "Are you kidding me?"

"No," he said quietly, "It's yours."

I was already crawling inside and inspecting the interior, trying out the steering wheel, cranking it up. Dad had even included a full tank of gas, I noticed. I got out to hug him, and then he handed me the payment booklet.

"Don't miss a payment or they'll come get it," he said as he slowly walked away.

I've been working ever since.

In college, I had three jobs to help pay for school bills. One was at a local fast food restaurant. That was my meal plan all four years. The second was at a local trucking company. It was the best paying job I had while I was in college, but it was an all-night shift. For the third job, I was the janitor at a local church. It paid peanuts. A few years later, however, that church hired me as part of the pastoral staff, so I made a lateral move over to associate pastor. All of you with ministry experience will get that joke.

I was on the full-time staff at the church for five years, and then Cheryl and I applied for missionary appointment. We were approved in 1989, left for language school in Costa Rica in 1990, and arrived in Honduras in 1991, where we lived and served until 2002. We came back to the states and worked as campus chaplains at a local university, with some part-time subbing on the side at a private academy. In 2006, I became part of the full-time staff at the academy and that's where I've been ever since.

I know that's a lot of moving around, changing countries, and changing jobs, but basically I've done the same thing for each of the various organizations which employed me: I have been a teacher. It's not a flashy profession or a lucrative one, but it has proven to be extremely fulfilling for me, whether I was working with teenagers in that first church, adults in Costa Rica and Honduras, or university and high school students here in the Charlotte area. I say all this to make a point.

If Parkinson's causes me to have to give up teaching sooner rather than later, I will be devastated. I cannot see that happening any time soon, based on my symptoms now and the effectiveness of my treatments. However, if my Parkinson's progresses to the moderate or advanced stages, I will have to make some gut-wrenching decisions.

~

Because the progression and severity of Parkinson's is different for each individual, the question of whether you should continue to work varies from person to person, as well. Generally speaking, I believe you should work for as long as you are able, and I think this for a variety of reasons, not the least of which is that work is built into our DNA. Even if you are set financially, you should find a place to put your talents to use. We call that volunteering.

The benefits of working are numerous, but perhaps one of the most important is that, for many of us, our sense of self-worth comes from our jobs. In an article in *USA Today* a few years ago entitled "At Work: Job, self-esteem tied tightly together," psychotherapist Charles Allen stated: "Self-esteem and self-worth are closely aligned with working. When you have a job, you have a continuous source of feedback that you are a contributing member of society…. . You feel it in the depths of your brain." I like that phrase.

The opposite is also true. Many of those who are

unemployed tend to be depressed. In the same article, Psychotherapist Jonathan Alpert describes them as usually feeling hopeless and helpless, their sense of identity greatly diminished. "Employment provides a sense of purpose … of belongingness. Those who are unemployed lack that purpose," says Alpert.

I suppose that everyone who retires must go through some of those same feelings. At the church I worked in during college, the senior pastor came out of retirement to take over our little thirty-five-member church, and he grew it to around 600 or 700 in attendance. The church went from nearly closing its doors in bankruptcy to a position of financial strength. When the pastor stepped down to re-retire years later, we all honored him and spoke of his noble willingness to forego his first retirement for the sake of the church. Then, his wife revealed the truth: "I was just so glad that church got him out of the house for several hours a day all these years. Before that, he was depressed and driving me crazy!"

Recently, I had the privilege of meeting former astronaut Rich Clifford and his wife, Nancy, at one of the premier showings of a documentary based on his life, *The Astronaut's Secret*. The film is about how Rich and NASA kept the secret that Rich had been diagnosed with Parkinson's as he was preparing for his last shuttle mission. NASA decided to let him go, anyway, because it did not seem to interfere with his duties, nor put anyone else on the flight at risk. They kept the decision a secret, so the press wouldn't make the flight all about Parkinson's. Now, after seventeen years, Rich is telling his story. In person, he seemed to be a very friendly but quiet man who was having to get used to the spotlight again—now not only as an American hero but as a hero among the Parkinson's community as well. What I liked most was when he and his wife were talking about his recent retirement. His version was different from Nancy's version. I asked Nancy how she felt about all the togetherness they were experiencing. She smiled and whispered, "Thank goodness for golf!"

"Oh, you both play?" I asked.

She said, "No, just him, and it usually takes him all morning."

I'm beginning to see a pattern here, aren't you?

Retiring at the right age is one thing, no matter how much the spouses already at home may miss their free time. However, it's a whole different story if you aren't quite ready to retire or even close to that age, and Parkinson's is one of the reasons you even have to consider it. The loss of identity and lack of purpose that comes with leaving the workforce should be weighed as we make our decisions.

I like the two questions that NASA asked: Does Parkinson's interfere with your duties or the mission? Does Parkinson's put you or anyone else at risk on the job? If the answer is *no* to both of those questions, then my vote would be to stay with your job and embrace the feeling of belonging, the positive feedback, and the sense of purpose. If the answer is *yes* to either one of those questions, then you do have some decisions to make.

Let's go with the former possibility first: You are able to say no to both questions. Then, by all means, stay employed. That's what my friend Dave did. He was diagnosed eleven years ago and from that day until now, he has held down a full-time job.

Over coffee at Panera, he told me: "I could easily have stayed home, wallowed in my depression, vented my deeply felt anger, and just vegged out watching television all day. After all, there are 3,000 plus channels now. Surely, I would have found something worth watching. But I needed to keep doing the work, so I could stay sharp mentally and stay connected socially, as opposed to isolating myself, which is a real temptation and tendency for those of us with Parkinson's."

Dave credits his decision to continue working with being the main reason he is still doing so well cognitively and physically. Well, that and the DBS surgery he had two and a half years ago. But he had already done eight and a half years before the surgery, so his decision to have the DBS done just enhanced his ability to do his job.

Dave did confess one more extenuating circumstance that kept him employed. He said, "My wife and I had budgeted for retirement based on two incomes. If we cut that down to just her salary when I was only forty-six, then we wouldn't have made our financial goals. I know not everyone with Parkinson's has that option, but I did and I chose to continue working. It was the best decision I could have made."

Another good friend also talked about the financial part of the decision. Hart, who was diagnosed with Parkinson's six years ago, explained that a primary reason he stayed in the workforce was because he felt a need to pay his bills. His remarks reminded me of the scene from the Christmas classic, *It's A Wonderful Life*, in which George Bailey (played by Jimmy Stewart) is talking with the angel Clarence (played by Henry Travers). Clarence has just explained that he is George's guardian angel, so George asks him, "Don't happen to have 8,000 bucks on you, do you?" When Clarence replies that they don't use money in heaven, George replies with one of my favorite lines in the whole movie: "Well, it comes in pretty handy down here, bub!" We all know that reality, some of us more than others.

Yet, Hart, like Dave, points to an even greater need in his life, the need to be productive. He believes the more effort we put toward that end, the greater the sense of achievement, whether you get compensated or not. So, he continues to serve as an associate pastor, visiting and teaching on a regular basis. He admits that sometimes the tremor in his right hand wants its own sideshow. He tries to rest it on the pulpit or clamp it to his chest under his folded arm. For obvious reasons, he cannot hold it in front, and it looks equally awkward behind his back. He appears to be scratching. But he doesn't want to give up speaking in front of people. "That would be taking away an opportunity to be productive," he says.

Hart is also quite the handyman, and he enjoys taking on home improvement projects. The problem, once again, is the tremor sideshow. Ever the pastor, he says that the shaking hand reminds him of Romans 7:15: "I do not understand what I do. For what I want to do I do not do, but what I hate I do." He likes to quote Winston Churchill's famous quip: "Never, never, never give up!" Continuing to work and produce is his way of showing that, with God's help, even this challenging diagnosis of Parkinson's can have a positive side to it. As Hart says: "Our job is to find that positive side!"

But let's also look at the other possibility, the one where you have to answer *yes* to one or both of those NASA questions. If Parkinson's puts you or anyone else at risk on the job, then it's an easy call. We simply must choose to step away for the well being of all concerned. I think that's what Rich Clifford would have done on that shuttle mission. It's what I had to do on a slightly less significant job: activities bus driver for the academy where I teach. OK, it's way less significant than a shuttle mission.

After my first two daughters graduated from the school, I had one daughter still at home with four years of high school left. She played volleyball for the academy and, so I could attend all her games, I got my CDL—commercial driver's license. Then, I volunteered to drive the team bus. It probably was not very cool to have your dad drive you to all the games, but I never missed an opportunity if I could help it. The chance to go to the volleyball games, that is, not to make her feel uncool. Well, maybe it was a little of both.

Because of that CDL, I also became the most popular chaperone for all the school's trips: the lower school field trips, the annual junior class trip to Charleston, the seniors-only night at retreat, and the annual senior trip—which back in those days was a week-long cruise. I got invited to them all because I was the one male chaperone who also happened to be licensed to drive the activity bus.

At the time I was diagnosed with Parkinson's four years ago, the Federal Department of Transportation required me to come in every year for a physical to prove that I was still capable of driving. All other CDL holders came in once every two years. I didn't mind the extra check-up. They were just doing their due diligence. However, this past year, the policy changed. On the back of the form that we always filled out, they now had a list of disqualifying conditions and circumstances. Guess what was near the top of the list? At first, I wanted to appeal the new decision that seemed so arbitrarily handed down. But when I had cooled off a little bit, I realized that the school did not need to take on that kind of liability. Would I have wanted my daughters riding with someone with a potentially hazardous neurological condition? The answer, of course, is no.

It worked out extremely well for me in the end. I had made quite a reputation for myself as a super chaperone over the years, so I still got invited to go on the annual trips and eventually took over as planner of those trips, which meant I went every time. Hey, it's a tough life, but somebody has to do it. Only now, I get one of the other teachers with a CDL to do the driving. Wake me when we get there, will you?

Returning to the two NASA questions once more, there's one more scenario. What if Parkinson's does interfere with your duties? Nobody's life is put at risk, but the symptoms do sometimes keep you from doing your job well. In my first book, I talked about the fact that I often have to make adjustments in my classes or in our weekly chapel services, such as sitting down to teach instead of standing. If your place of employment will allow certain accommodations for you—that is, ways to work around your symptoms—and you can still fulfill your duties and serve the business well, then that's a win-win for all concerned.

Someone who has lived out that exact set of circumstances is my good friend, Maureen. She and her husband, Ben, joined my support group about eight months ago. They had just moved to Charlotte from New Mexico to be near their son and, hopefully, some eventual grandchildren. Of course, the son has to find a wife first. No pressure, right? I think the first day they visited our support group, they asked how they could help me. I liked them from the start.

As I came to know them, Maureen confided that her greatest fear when she was first diagnosed with Parkinson's was that she would not be able to continue working. She had been an interior designer for forty years, and she was not ready to quit. Besides, it isn't work when your heart is in it. She summed up her attitude: "When you love doing something and you have a passion for it, you're just getting paid to have fun."

The first year after Maureen's diagnosis in New

Mexico, her dosages weren't right, her symptoms weren't managed well, and the side effects from the medications were worse than the symptoms. To even keep working that first year was a challenge, and she decided to change neurologists.

Maureen found a movement disorder specialist the second time around who changed her meds. There was an immediate and profound difference: "I felt like myself again. The usual visual effects of Parkinson's disappeared, and I was left with the not-so-obvious ones such as digestive problems, sleep problems, and so on. At that point, most people were not even aware that I had anything wrong unless I told them." It has now been six years since her diagnosis, and her symptoms have remained constant. She hasn't had to increase dosages, and she doesn't experience any of the outward problems unless she gets off-schedule taking her meds.

When Maureen came to Charlotte, she began working full-time as a designer for a local home furnishings store. Immediately, fatigue was a new factor in the equation, so she asked her employer for an accommodation. Could she transfer to another store and work part-time? The store was more than happy to make the change. She would now do four days a week and have weekends and Wednesdays free. With this adjustment, as she put it, she's off and running. She feels better, she's writing up more sales working part-time than she ever did as a full-timer, and she loves her work. Plus, she gets to see her son more and bug him about those grandchildren.

Maureen, by the way, is ... well, old enough to retire if she wanted to, but she doesn't want to. When she first found her movement disorder specialist, Maureen asked her about continuing to work. Her doctor had told her that as long as she felt like it, she should work as much as she could. The more she worked, the longer she would be able to work and the better she would feel.

"That has certainly been the case for me," Maureen said proudly. "I will continue to work as long as I can. It keeps the brain functioning."

I asked her husband, Ben, how he felt about her continuing to work. He told me, "Maureen has a very strong will that allows her to rise to the occasion when necessary. That's why she has been able to keep working." He also believes that her strong will has been a major factor in how she has been able to deal with Parkinson's in general. "Besides," he whispered to me, "when I mentioned one time that maybe she shouldn't push as hard as she once did, both she and the doctor totally disagreed with me. The doctor said that Maureen would be the best judge of what she was capable of doing and what she was not. That system has worked out pretty well for the both of us."

Then, there's my Parkinson's buddy, Vince. I call him my Parkinson's buddy because we work at the same academy and we highly suspect that someone there has contaminated the water supply, although we have been unable to prove that conspiracy theory. He has been diagnosed for seven years, as opposed to my four years, but we started our support group as co-facilitators and often get together to discuss the ins-and-outs and ups-and-downs of life with Parkinson's. He's a good friend.

At work, however, Vince has been gradually dropping a class from his load every other year or so, and two years ago, he and his wife—both math geniuses—officially switched places. He took the part-time teaching load, and she took over the full-time load. Accommodations were made for him. He was able to sit down to teach when he needed to, like I do, and I believe everyone is completely understanding of his condition, as they are with mine.

"However," he explains, "I make more mistakes than I used to when I explain problems on the board, and I don't like when that happens. Quite frankly, I don't know if the culprit is related to Parkinson's or simply old age, but my one mistake could lead the students not to understand a topic and that misunderstanding could in turn lead to a greater confusion later. Ultimately, my mistakes could affect a child's grade or worse, their enjoyment of math." That would be the ultimate negative outcome, Vince would argue.

He says, "My symptoms affect every minute of my life. However, when they begin to affect a student's ability to learn—and his or her parents happen to be paying customers—is when I felt I should make those changes." The bottom line is that Vince has had to decide what his limitations are and how much those limitations are affecting his ability to teach the higher-level math courses. Of course, he has forgotten more math than I ever knew in the first place—not because of Parkinson's, mind you, but just because his brain is so full, he's probably running out of storage. I still think he's a genius. And geniuses get to choose when they want to drop a class.

By the way, they won't let me choose, yet. Hmm, I wonder why.

~

The decision to continue to work is personal and based on many factors. Sometimes, the decision is taken out of our hands by our doctors, our circumstances, or our employers. There is a line of defense with employers. It's called the Americans with Disabilities Act (ADA). Regarding the ADA, the Parkinson's Disease Foundation's website states:

By law, people with Parkinson's are protected under the ADA against discrimination in employment practices. This law requires employers to make reasonable accommodations for employees, as long as they do not impose an "undue hardship" on the employer's business. A reasonable accommodation is defined as "any modification or adjustment to a job or the work environment that will enable a qualified applicant or employee with a disability to participate in the application process or to perform essential job functions." (pdf.org/en/fall05_employment)

Of course, if the ADA has to be invoked, the question I would ask myself is: Do I really want to be associated with this kind of company, business, or employer? It may come down to a matter of principle for you, and if that's true, then I say go for it. Maybe you can be the one to help them see the light.

What I wish for everyone is what I have experienced. I came back to my place of employment and told my boss immediately that I had been diagnosed with Parkinson's. That was on a Friday. If I remember correctly, he got a little misty-eyed and said something to the effect that life is not fair and what in the world—I think he said *world*—was God thinking? He was already at the anger stage, and I hadn't even gotten out of denial yet. We let the leadership team know that afternoon, the rest of the faculty and staff on the following Monday, and all of the students in the upper grades on Wednesday of that same week.

Everybody prayed and shared words of encouragement in the beginning. Later, as my symptoms began to manifest themselves a little more and I became increasingly self-conscious about those embarrassing moments, both the faculty and students told me not to worry about those incidents. They all loved me, regardless. As I said before, teaching is not a very flashy profession, nor a lucrative one, but it has its rewards. At our school, there's a profound sense of family. I wish everyone could experience the level of acceptance that I have felt. I know that's unrealistic, but one can still hope.

As long as I am able, I want to continue to try to do the same duties with the same excellence and enthusiasm that I would have done them if I had not been diagnosed with Parkinson's. The result? The people where I work think I'm Superman—a Superman who shuffles, mind you—but a Superman, nonetheless. Again, I know that I am now in the mild stage of Parkinson's, and my cape and tights will eventually have to be retired. But for as long as I can work, I plan to do so.

Chapter Eight
Winning

*I press on toward the goal to win the prize for which God
has called me heavenward in Christ Jesus.*
—Philippians 3:14

When I was in third grade, I got a new bike. It wasn't
really new, just new to me. It was rescued from the local
junkyard. When we were growing up, most of our bikes
were rescues. Dad thought you lost too much in
depreciation the second you drove the new one off the lot.
Plus, he liked to work on things, build things, repair things,
recycle things, resurrect things. He was, and is, a jack-of-
all-trades and master of several. Just for the record, I got
none of his skills, but I did get a bike that third-grade year.
It was a beauty, or, at least, it became one.

The frame was a nice, rained-on, rusty color when we
picked it up. But that was just oxidation, my Dad had
explained. The frame was solid, the welds were sure. All it
needed was some paint. But first, we had to sand it down,
then recheck the welds. They don't make them like this
anymore, Dad had said. Then, we painted it royal blue
from stem to stern. Of course, we did have to buy some
new parts, such as the tires and chain, the cruiser

handlebars, and the most important piece of all: a royal blue banana seat with silver sparkles. Everybody on my street wanted a bike like mine, but Dad had no desire to open a bike shop. There were beehives to build, chicken coops to repair, and playhouses to roof—and we were burning daylight.

The Monday after the bike became mine, I rode it the two blocks to my elementary school and steered it toward the bike rack beside the third-grade door. We commuters had our own special place to park.

And then I saw it. One of my classmates had a brand new bike, too. But it wasn't a rescue. It was a three-speed touring bike, and it looked sleek, elegant, and fast.

"Wow, where did you get that?" I asked him.

He answered, "My mom and dad gave it to me Saturday, for no special reason. Uhhh ... where did you get yours?"

"The junkyard," I answered. I was innocent, little Opie Taylor, telling the truth. "My dad and I put it together this weekend. Look at that banana seat!" But I had given him all that he needed with the word *junkyard*.

"Oh, is that where your family does all their shopping?" he started teasing.

"Boys, come inside," the teacher intervened, standing at the door quietly. "You both have very nice bikes."

I beamed. He sneered. He was just getting started. For the rest of the morning, he made jokes about how my family went to the junkyard for everything: bikes, furniture, cars, clothing, and food. After lunch, he started in on the bikes. His was faster, nicer-looking, newer, cleaner. If we were in a race, he would leave me in the dust, kicking it into third gear and watching me pedal my little one-speed as hard as I could, miles behind him. My bike would probably fall apart, he said, since I had helped put it together. It wouldn't even make it around the track, he taunted. Too bad we couldn't go and prove it right now.

"Enough!" yelled my teacher. "Third grade, close your books. We're going outside." Everybody screamed and ran toward the door. They all knew what was about to take place. They had all gotten sick of the kid with the new bike and his comments whispered across the room all day long. As for me, I began to wonder if maybe the boy was right. Maybe my bike would fall apart as soon as we started around the track.

But my teacher was smarter than that. She looked out over the two acres of land the school had behind the buildings. The playground, baseball field, kickball field, and basketball courts were all close to the classrooms, and a dirt track circled all four areas. It wasn't an official track for running. The dirt track was just where the path had been worn bare by years and years of so many feet following the same paths to the same places every day.

"The track is too short for this important race," she said. "We need to go cross country. We need to prove once and for all which bike is faster. So, here's what we'll do. You both will go straight down the track between the kick ball field and the baseball field, but when it turns to the left, you keep heading for the edge of the field. At the big oak tree, turn left and go all the way to the corner of the field, then across the back side, and when you get to the fence on the other side, you'll come straight back here. First one through the monkey bars wins. Any questions?"

We both got on our bikes and waited for the signal.

"On your mark, get set, go!" shouted the teacher, and we took off. All the other kids started screaming. I later wondered if the teacher got into trouble for the race we had that day. I never heard if she did, but I didn't worry about such things in third grade. I was pedaling as hard as I could go. The boy with the new bike took the early lead. I didn't know how a three-speed worked, but I did notice in those first few seconds that he was pulling away. That ended as soon as we left the track. The playing field had been leveled, so to speak, as soon as we got out to the unleveled grassy areas of the open fields. We both were bouncing on our seats as we went over the ruts in the ground. By the time we got to the first turn, I had caught him. When we got to the second turn, the ground dipped low, and some water had accumulated. We saw the mud at the same time and I went flying through, but he was not so lucky. It was like a scene from a kids' movie, where the bad guy wipes out and falls into the mud. The rest was history. I cleared the third turn, just as he was getting up and walking his bike to the higher ground. As I started the straight stretch from the back corner to the monkey bars, it was like everything went into slow motion and we were back in the movie again. All the other kids were running toward me and yelling, "You won! You won!" and as I flew through the monkey bars, they were chasing after me, skipping and laughing as if they had all won the race, too. It was the best day of my life, at least up until third grade. OK, it might have been the best day in all of elementary school. In fact, I'm pretty sure that it was. It always feels good when you win.

~

I've been thinking a lot lately about what it looks like to win against Parkinson's. Recently, I was down in Spartanburg, South Carolina, and I attended the Victory Summit® sponsored by the Davis Phinney Foundation for Parkinson's. The one-day event is meant to inform and inspire those with Parkinson's and their loved ones to live well with the disease. It is a high-energy and thoroughly enjoyable way to spend a Saturday.

Davis Phinney was one of the cycling greats for nearly two decades. He was an Olympic bronze medalist in 1984, and he is one of only three U.S. cyclists to win multiple stages in the prestigious Tour de France bike race. When he retired from cycling in 1993, he had the most victories of any other U.S. cyclist in history, with 328 in all.

Seven years later he was diagnosed with young onset Parkinson's disease, although he had manifest symptoms for years before the official diagnosis came. In his book, *The Happiness of Pursuit*, he admits to going through a dark place in his life in the beginning, but things turned around when he realized that there were ways to maintain a high quality of life, despite the disease. He started the Davis Phinney Foundation to promote a more proactive approach to dealing with Parkinson's.

The Davis Phinney Foundation's one-day seminars, as I mentioned, are called The Victory Summit® events, and they are all about celebrating the everyday wins, smart decisions, and positive attitudes of the people that are doing things right. The program that day started with a session entitled "Building a Parkinson's Toolkit," in which the speaker promoted treatment awareness, exercise, nutrition, emotional well-being and putting together a support team. That was followed by talks on the "The Power of Movement" and "Enhancing Quality of Life." Are you starting to see the theme here?

Throughout the day, there were various movement breaks during which we did speech therapy and gentle yoga exercises, along with our 600 fellow attendees. They also celebrated two local heroes with Parkinson's from that geographical area who had served the needs of others within the Parkinson's community. The day ended with a pep talk from Davis Phinney himself in which he spoke on the moments of victory we should be celebrating every day.

I didn't record his exact words from the speech, but in the manual entitled "Every Victory Counts®" offered to everyone in attendance, Phinney wrote these words:

> I learned much about myself through years of competing successfully in tough, demanding events. I came to understand the importance of focus and purpose; that paying attention to and being engaged in the process is just as important as the achievement of the goals. I came to understand that victory—that elusive, electric moment of triumph—was not exclusive to those who crossed the finish line first. These are lessons that are rooted in me, and they help me now in the much more challenging race called Parkinson's disease. This race, a no-holds-barred winner-take-all type of event, demands everything from me. Let down my guard, and it'll knock me flat—but by refusing to give in, by exercising daily, by eating well and most especially, by maintaining a positive attitude—I find ways to win.

I was impressed with the whole event, from start to finish. When we left, most of us felt better about ourselves than we had when we arrived. I think that was the Davis Phinney Foundation's goal from the start. I, for one, believe they succeeded.

I had met Davis Phinney the night before at the volunteers' appreciation dinner. He and his wife, Connie, were making the rounds to each table. I even had my photograph taken with him. I noticed that he looked exhausted that evening, his words came out slowly, and he was dragging a little bit physically. In other words, he looked exactly like I do many evenings. That was a real encouragement to me. Despite what he was feeling, he was plugging on, regardless. I do that, too. It was just nice to see that I wasn't the only one who struggled.

Did you catch the title of his book? *The Happiness of Pursuit.* It's an obvious play on the phrase, "the pursuit of happiness," from the U.S. Declaration of Independence, which states: "We hold these truths to be self-evident, that all men are created equal, that they are endowed by their Creator with certain unalienable Rights, that among these are Life, Liberty and the pursuit of Happiness." Phinney changed the order to emphasize that happiness can also be found in the pursuit itself. In other words, happiness is not just the destination; it's also what we can experience along the way.

The verse that topped the first page of this chapter has a similar message. Actually, to fully understand what Paul was trying to say here, we need to back up several verses and catch the whole context. This is what he wrote:

> But whatever were gains to me I now consider loss for the sake of Christ. What is more, I consider everything a loss because of the surpassing worth of knowing Christ Jesus my Lord, for whose sake I have lost all things. I consider them garbage, that I may gain Christ and be found in him, not having a righteousness of my own that comes from the law, but that which is through faith in Christ—the righteousness that comes from God on the basis of faith. I want to know Christ—yes, to know the power of his resurrection and participation in his sufferings, becoming like him in his death, and so, somehow, attaining to the resurrection from the dead (Philippians 3:7-11).

Not that I have already obtained all this, or have already arrived at my goal, but I press on to take hold of that for which Christ Jesus took hold of me. Brothers and sisters, I do not consider myself yet to have taken hold of it. But one thing I do: Forgetting what is behind and straining toward what is ahead, I press on toward the goal to win the prize for which God has called me heavenward in Christ Jesus" (Philippians 3:12-14).

Paul often used athletic analogies, sometimes just a word or phrase, as in 1 Timothy 6:12, and sometimes more lengthy ones, such as in 1 Corinthians 9:24-27. The phrase "press on" is a runner's term. It meant "to run swiftly in order to catch something or someone, or in order to reach a finish line or goal." He uses it the first time in verse 12 where he admits: "Not that I have already obtained all this, or have already arrived at my goal, but I press on to take hold of that for which Christ Jesus took hold of me."

Paul's running toward a goal, but he has not yet arrived, so he has to keep pushing; he has to keep pumping those legs; he has to keep up the pursuit. On this side of the goal, that's what it's all about: To never stop running. So, what was the goal anyway? What was waiting for him at the end of the race that made the pursuit so worthwhile? I think it's pretty obvious when you read verses 7-11. The goal was not a *what*, it was a *who*—Christ himself.

"All my past accomplishments," he says, "I now consider loss or garbage for the sake of Christ." His top priority, his aim, his goal was Christ himself: to know him, to gain him, to be found in him, to have a righteousness through faith in him, even to become like him in his death. "Nothing else matters. Everything else is secondary. I want Christ," Paul declares. "And I'm not going to stop pressing on until I reach my goal, until I reach him."

If you pause here and think about who is saying these words, it's really an incredible story. It's a 180-degree turn from the direction he was heading with his life. After all, this was the guy who had set out to destroy the church. He literally went from house to house, dragging off both men and women and putting them in prison. He had approved of the killing of Stephen, the first Christian martyr, and then took his murderous campaign of persecution on the road to cities beyond Jerusalem, looking to round up all the disciples of Jesus he possibly could (see Acts 8:1-3, 9:1-2). Of course, back then his name was Saul. He later changed his name to Paul, but it was the same person.

But there's a little play on words when you compare Philippians 3 and Acts 9. The Greek word translated "press on" in Philippians 3 is the same word translated "persecute" in Acts 9. So, when Paul has the life-changing, career-altering encounter with Jesus on the road to Damascus in Acts 9, the question that Jesus asks him is this one: "Saul, Saul, why do you *persecute* me?" Or put another way: "Why do you press on and run swiftly after me?" This might be where Paul got the term in the first place.

Then Paul responds: "Who are you, Lord?" His question makes it sound like he already knew the answer, don't you think?

"I am Jesus, whom you are persecuting," Jesus says again, or he could have worded it this way: "I am Jesus, the one you are pressing on after." From that day forward, Paul would press on in pursuit of Jesus but in a positive way.

Returning to Philippians 3, the second time he uses the phrase "press on" is verses 13-14: "Brothers and sisters, I do not consider myself yet to have taken hold of it. But one thing I do: Forgetting what is behind and straining toward what is ahead, I press on toward the goal to win the prize for which God has called me heavenward in Christ Jesus."

Again, Paul reiterates: "I'm not there yet. I'm still in pursuit." But if "pressing on" is the *what*, Paul now explains the *how*, with two key phrases: "forgetting what is behind" and "straining toward what is ahead." I think all great runners have to practice these two disciplines. The first has to do with letting go of whatever hardships or failures he or she has had to go through to get where they are now. Dwelling on the past is distracting to today's race. The same would be true of whatever victories or successes he or she has experienced. All that has happened up to now has to be forgotten in order to concentrate on the task at hand. In Paul's case, he's got to let go of his guilt and shame over his former sins; perhaps the hardest of all to forget will be the ones he committed against the followers of Christ themselves. But if God has forgiven him, then he must do so, too. Paul also has to let go of the former glories he enjoyed. None of that will help him in the race in which he finds himself now.

Instead of looking back, then, Paul needs to be facing forward and using all his energy and effort in finishing the race he's running. One can almost see the image of a runner leaning forward and with everything that he or she has within them, digging deep for that last burst of speed and endurance to cross the finish line first.

The writer of Hebrews talks about a race as well: "And let us run with perseverance the race marked out for us, fixing our eyes on Jesus, the pioneer and perfecter of faith" (Hebrews 12:1-2). It seems that there is one person who has already run the race—successfully, I might add—and now awaits us at the finish line: Jesus himself. It looks like Paul is going to get what he's been hoping for. It's no wonder he's straining toward what is ahead. Again, the *what* is a *who*.

Paul ends with these words: "I press on toward the goal to win the prize for which God has called me heavenward in Christ Jesus." So, now, there's a goal and a prize. What's the prize? Some would say heaven itself is the reward. And while it does sound like a beautiful place—there's no more death, mourning, crying or pain, for starters—it does not appear to be what Paul is talking about here. Heavenward is the direction he's going, but it's not the prize of this verse. It has to be something else.

Others say it might be the crowns we receive upon arrival in heaven. There are several possibilities mentioned in the Bible, the crown that will last forever (1 Corinthians 9:25), the victor's crown (2 Timothy 2:5), the crown of righteousness (2 Timothy 4:8), the crown of life (James 1:12), and the crown of glory (1 Peter 5:4). That would be a nice prize, one or more of those crowns. But again, that doesn't seem to fit because all the crowns seem to end up at the foot of the throne of the One who lives forever (Revelation 4:10).

Still others would say it's simply God's approval of a life well lived, as Jesus describes in Matthew 25. The story is often referred to as "The Parable of the Talents." The talents were really bags of gold. A man going on a journey entrusts his wealth to his servants. To one he gives five bags of gold, to another two bags, and to yet another one bag. While the master is away, the man who got five bags of gold goes out and earns five more bags. The man with two bags of gold gains two more. The third guy does not do as well. In fact, he does nothing.

Then, the master returns and checks on each man's success. To the first two men, he says what all of us want to hear when we get to heaven: "Well done, good and faithful servant! You have been faithful with a few things; I will put you in charge of many things. Come and share your master's happiness" (Matthew 25:21-22). Again, the third guy does not fare so well, but I'll let you read the rest of the story on your own. Everyone who heard Jesus tell the story knew which servants they wanted to emulate. But once more, I don't think that's the prize for Paul.

His reward, as he has stated all along, is Christ alone. Heaven sounds wonderful, the crowns would be meaningful, the words "Well done!" would be a delight to hear, but all that fails compared to the surpassing glory of just finally being with Jesus. He is both the goal and the prize. And he's the one that makes the lifelong pursuit worth it all.

I watched a race recently where the winner, a female runner who was yards ahead of everyone else, fell into the arms of her coach as she crossed the finish line. According to the commentator, that's how she ended every race, with her coach waiting on her and cheering her on until the very last step, at which point he would catch her as she collapsed from sheer exhaustion, leaving everything on the track. She won almost every race in which she ran, but the smile on her face seemed less about the winning and more about who was waiting across the finish line. I think Paul would have known exactly what she was experiencing.

~

So, what does it look like to win against Parkinson's? Well, if someone finds a cure, that would certainly be a win. I like the Michael J. Fox Foundation's single, urgent goal: Eliminate Parkinson's disease in our lifetime. I'm 100 percent behind that goal!

But what does winning look like short of a cure? I think it looks like getting up every day and saying, "Today I am determined to beat my Parkinson's!" and if at the end of the day you had any success at that whatsoever, then you count those little and big victories and put them in the win column. It's what Davis Phinney says at every one of his Victory Summits®: Every Victory Counts!

So, what counts as a victory? I beat Parkinson's every day that I walk 10,000 steps. That's my newest craze: a Fitbit. Mine is a simple Charge that counts the steps I take, the miles I walk, and the flights of stairs I climb. My daily goals are 10,000, five, and ten, respectively. I got the watch-like apparatus for my birthday this year, and every day since I've been walking my 10,000 steps. I'm currently forty-two days in a row with that count, and a friend recently challenged me to do 100, so 100 days it is. I cannot pass on a challenge.

I do most of my walking in the mornings, and if you could see my first fifteen to twenty minutes, you would see the fastest shuffler on the block. You would also hear me coming from a mile away. I sound like I'm sanding the sidewalks. After that initial time of adjustment, however, my legs limber up, and I start to get some flexibility, and I look like a normal walker. That's usually about the time the sun is coming up, so most of my shuffling is done in the dark. The neat thing about the Fitbit is that it tells me when I'm close and it vibrates when I hit my goal. If I go over my 10,000-step goal, it even gets a little sarcastic and calls me an overachiever. I like that!

I also beat Parkinson's every day that I volunteer for the Parkinson Association of the Carolinas! Whether that's with my support group at the local YMCA once a month— well, now twice a month since we added a game day for all of us just to sit down and play cards together—or as a member of one of the PAC committees that serve our Parkinson's community here in the Carolinas. I was temporarily assigned to two different committees, Awareness and Support Services, but I conveniently forgot to step off one of them when the time came. That's because I love being involved and helping in every way I can.

I just got an email from PAC this week asking me to help put together what we're going to call Support Group in a Box, a resource kit for anyone who wants to start a Parkinson's support group in their community. We want to give them all the materials they could possibly need to lead their group effectively and for the long haul. I love the fact that I have Parkinson's and I get to serve others who have to deal with this disease, too.

I beat Parkinson's every day that I take a nature walk with my grandson. I started last summer when I was out pushing him around in the stroller, and we took a few photographs of flowers, ducks, squirrels—whatever we saw! Well, those little walks have developed quite a following in our social media world. I have two rules for a photograph to be legit. Elisha has to be in the picture and so does the animal, plant, or scene we are trying to capture.

One of the first ones was simply Elisha pointing to a red flower and saying, "Wait, let's stop and smell the roses." One of the latest ones showed Elisha pointing to a mother duck and her babies, and saying "Papa, make way for ducklings!" I think we've posted 107 so far with no plans to stop any time soon.

All of these things may seem small or trivial to outsiders, but for those who know anything about Parkinson's, they represent victories worth counting. And I do count them … and others.

I beat Parkinson's every day that I go to work and teach high school students.

I beat Parkinson's every day that I get to dance with my wife.

I beat Parkinson's every day that I get to Skype with my daughters, no matter where they happen to be in the world.

I beat Parkinson's every day that I play cards with my friends.

I beat Parkinson's every day that I write another chapter in a book.

I beat Parkinson's every day that I wash the dishes, do the laundry, or vacuum the house. Well, maybe not the vacuuming.

I beat Parkinson's every day that I enjoy a good movie.

I beat Parkinson's every day that I do the grocery shopping.

I beat Parkinson's every day that I visit a friend in the hospital, even if I am moving more slowly than the patient.

I beat Parkinson's every day that I don't quit or say I'm done.

I beat Parkinson's every day that I shuffle on.

I beat Parkinson's every day that I help someone else shuffle on. In fact, that's when I really beat Parkinson's … when it's two against one.

Acknowledgments

First of all, to Cheryl: You are my good thing and I am so glad I found you. And that you asked me to that Sadie Hawkins event. Oops, was I supposed to share that? "I'm thinking that it must be you, all of my life."

To Brittany, Lauren, Sarah and Elisha: Three great kids and one grandkid. I'm so proud of the wonderfulness of each one of you. "I will always love you true, no matter what you say or do."

To DeLonn: I am grateful for the "random" phone call that led me to so many blessings, including the completion of my degree and this book. Thank you for the encouraging push in the right direction.

To Dr. Englert: Thank you for your kindness, care, and friendship through all of this, for answering all my questions and for always making me feel like I am your only patient. Oh, yeah, and for not holding a grudge. (Wink, wink.)

To Kristen and Tim: Thank you for this second go-around, this time with two kids in the house. You do such quality work, it's worth the wait. Is it too soon to tell you that I'm thinking of a third?

To God: I still believe in the reality of you, no matter what my circumstances happen to be. I still believe in your promises, even when I do not see every one of them come to fruition in my life. I still believe in you, God, even when I don't understand it all. I still believe ...

CPSIA information can be obtained
at www.ICGtesting.com
Printed in the USA
LVOW10s1514030517
533132LV00008B/635/P